CASE STUDIES *in* PATIENT SAFETY

Foundations for Core Competencies

Julie K. Johnson, MSPH, PhD

Professor
Department of Surgery
Center for Healthcare Studies
Institute for Public Health and Medicine
Feinburg School of Medicine
Northwestern University
Chicago, Illinois

Helen W. Haskell, MA

President
Mothers Against Medical Error
Columbia, South Carolina

Paul R. Barach, MD, MPH

Guest Professor
School of Medicine
University of Oslo
Oslo, Norway

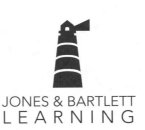

JONES & BARTLETT
LEARNING

World Headquarters
Jones & Bartlett Learning
5 Wall Street
Burlington, MA 01803
978-443-5000
info@jblearning.com
www.jblearning.com

Jones & Bartlett Learning books and products are available through most bookstores and online booksellers. To contact Jones & Bartlett Learning directly, call 800-832-0034, fax 978-443-8000, or visit our website, www.jblearning.com.

Substantial discounts on bulk quantities of Jones & Bartlett Learning publications are available to corporations, professional associations, and other qualified organizations. For details and specific discount information, contact the special sales department at Jones & Bartlett Learning via the above contact information or send an email to specialsales@jblearning.com.

Production Credits

VP, Executive Publisher: David Cella	Manufacturing and Inventory Control Supervisor:
Publisher: Michael Brown	Amy Bacus
Associate Editor: Lindsey Mawhiney	Composition: Cenveo Publisher Services
Associate Production Editor: Rebekah Linga	Cover Design: Kristin E. Parker
Art Development Editor: Joanna Lundeen	Rights and Photo Research Coordinator: Mary Flatley
Art Development Assistant: Shannon Sheehan	Cover Image: © Stockbyte/Thinkstock
Senior Marketing Manager:	Printing and Binding: Edwards Brothers Malloy
Sophie Fleck Teague	Cover Printing: Edwards Brothers Malloy

Library of Congress Cataloging-in-Publication Data
Johnson, Julie K., author.
 Case studies in patient safety : foundations for core competencies / Julie Johnson, Helen Haskell, and Paul Barach.
  p. ; cm.
 Includes bibliographical references and index.
 ISBN 978-1-4496-8154-8 (paper)
 I. Haskell, Helen, author. II. Barach, Paul, author. III. Title.
 [DNLM: 1. Patient Safety–Case Reports. 2. Clinical Competence–Case Reports. 3. Medical Errors–prevention & control–Case Reports. 4. Quality of Health Care–Case Reports. WX 185]
 R859.7.S43
 610.28'9–dc23
                                   2014038075

6048

Printed in the United States of America
19 18 17 16 15   10 9 8 7 6 5 4 3 2 1

Dedication

We dedicate this book to the memory of
Lewis Wardlaw Haskell Blackman, a shining light
extinguished far too soon.

CONTENTS

Contributors   *vii*

Acknowledgments   *xiii*

Foreword   *xv*

Preface   *xxi*

Introduction   *xxv*

Section I: Patient Care   **1**

1   It's Hard to Kill a Healthy 15-Year-Old   5
2   Routine Appendectomy   15
3   The Origins of the Mid Staffordshire Inquiry into
    the National Health Service   29
4   Consent and Disclosure in Pediatric Heart Surgery   47

Section II: Knowledge for Practice   **61**

5   I'm Left in Fear: An Account of Harm in Maternity Care   63
6   A Routine Endoscopic Procedure   73
7   The Last Run: An Undiagnosed Heart Rhythm Disturbance   83

Section III: Practice-Based Learning and Improvement   **97**

8   Improving Care for People with Intellectual Disability   101
9   A Cascade of Small Events: Learning from an Unexpected
    Postsurgical Death   117
10 Accidental Fall in a Hospital   129

Section IV: Interpersonal and Communication Skills   **141**

11 Not Considered a Partner: A Mother's Story of a Tonsillectomy
    Gone Wrong   143
12 Lost: A Patient's Search for Answers for Intractable Pain   153
13 The Silence of the Hospital: Lessons on Supporting Patients
    and Staff After an Adverse Event   163

Section V: Professionalism   **175**

14 The Big Picture: A Terminally Ill Patient in a Fragmented System 177
15 Without a Heart: The Legal Sequelae of an Unexplained

Hospital Death   191
16   Small Steps: From Medication Adjustment to Permanent Disability   209
17   The Definition of Alive: The Story of an Equivocal Birth   219

Section VI: Systems-Based Practice   *229*

18   Not for IV Use: The Story of an Enteral Tubing Misconnection   231
19   Death Despite Known Drug Allergy   247
20   The Trial Meant for You: The Lifelong Medical Journey
     of a Child with a Complex Congenital Condition   261

Section VII: Interprofessional Collaboration   *273*

21   Failure to Rescue   277
22   Unmonitored: A Postsurgical Narcotic Overdose in the Hospital   287
23   The Voice That Is Missing: A Mother's Journey
     in Patient Safety Advocacy   297
24   When Healing Harms: Recovering from a Multisystem
     Traumatic Injury   309

Section VIII: Personal and Professional Development   *321*

Afterword Personal and Professional Development   323
Appendix   Recommended List of Core Competencies
               for Health Professions   327

Index   *333*

Diana Arachi, MPH, MA, BA (Hons), Cert PMP
University of New South Wales
Sydney, NSW, Australia

Julie Bailey, CBE
Founder, Cure the NHS
Worcester, England

Carolyn Canfield
Citizen-patient
Honorary Lecturer
Department of Family Medicine
Faculty of Medicine
The University of British Columbia
Vancouver, BC Canada

Linda Carswell
Director, Jerry Carswell Memorial Foundation
Houston, TX, USA

Dr. Bruce Chenoweth
Senior Developmental Psychiatrist
Kogarah Developmental Disability Service
Metro-Regional Intellectual Disability Network
St George Hospital
South Eastern Sydney Local Health District

Conjoint Senior Clinical Lecturer, School of Psychiatry
University of New South Wales
Sydney, NSW, Australia

Deborah Debono, RN, RM, BA
Centre for Healthcare Resilience and Implementation Science
Australian Institute of Health Innovation
Macquarie University
Sydney, NSW, Australia

Dale R. Ford, MBBS, FRACGP, FACRRM
Principal Clinical Advisor, Improvement Foundation
Australia Greater Health Warrnambool
Hamilton, Victoria, Australia

John James, PhD, DABT
Founder, Patient Safety America
NASA Chief Toxicologist (Retired)
Houston, TX, USA

Meg Harrison Humphrey
Houston, TX, USA

Linda Kenney
MITSS (Medically Induced Trauma Support Services)
Chestnut Hill, MA, USA

Robert Leitner, MBBS, FRACP
Developmental Paediatrician
Director, Kogarah Developmental Assessment Service
Metro-Regional Intellectual Disability Network
St. George Hospital
South Eastern Sydney Local Health District
Sydney, NSW, Australia

Janet Long, BSc (Hons), MN, PhD
John Walsh Centre for Rehabilitation Research
University of Sydney
Sydney, NSW, Australia

Tanya Lord, MPH, PhD
Patient Engagement Consultant
Nashua, NH, USA

Nicola Mackintosh, RN, BSc, MSc, PhD
Research Fellow
Division of Women's Health, School of Medicine
King's College London, UK

Farah Magrabi, BE, PhD
Associate Professor
Australian Institute of Health Innovation
Macquarie University
Sydney, NSW, Australia

Mary Ellen Mannix, MRPE
Founder, James's Project
Wayne, PA, USA

Kirsten Morrise
Salt Lake City, UT, USA

Lisa Morrise, MArts
Co-Lead Partnership for Patients PFE Affinity Group
LAM Professional Services, LLC
Salt Lake City, UT, USA

Sandra Pintabona, RN
Perth, Western Australia, Australia

Susanna Rance, PhD
Visiting Research Associate
King's College
London, UK
Senior Research Fellow
Plymouth University Peninsula
Schools of Medicine and Dentistry
Plymouth, UK

Glenda Rodgers, RNC, BSN
Legal Nurse Consultant
Troy, KS, USA

Jane Sandall, PhD, MSc, BSc (Hons), RM, RN, HV
Professor of Social Science and Women's Health
King's College
London, UK

David Skalicky, MBBS, FAFRM
Rehabilitation Physician
Northern Intellectual Disability Health
Sydney, NSW, Australia

Karen Sterner
Bastrop, TX, USA

Kathy Torpie, MS
Psychologist, International Healthcare Speaker and Patient
    Experience Advisor
www.kathytorpie.com
Auckland, New Zealand

Laura Batz Townsend
Louise H. Batz Patient Safety Foundation
Austin, TX, USA

Linda Ward
Bastrop, TX, USA

Kylie Watson, BSc, BM, MSc
Research Associate
King's Patient Safety and Service Quality Research Centre
London, UK
Senior Midwife and Supervisor of Midwives
Central Manchester University Hospitals
Foundation NHS Trust
Manchester, UK

Jurgen Wille
Senior Social Worker
Kogarah Developmental Assessment Service
Metro-Regional Intellectual Disability Network
St. George Hospital
South Eastern Sydney Local Health District
Sydney, NSW, Australia

Helena Williams, MBBS, FRACGP
Executive Clinical Director
Southern Adelaide-Fleurieu-Kangaroo
   Island Medicare Local Limited
Blackwood, SA, Australia

ACKNOWLEDGMENTS

This book has been a multi-year journey, and we greatly appreciate the encouragement and support from colleagues, friends, and family. We have particularly benefited from the feedback of Drs. Arnold Kaluzny, Paul Batalden, and David Leach, who provided insight and understanding of the importance of making this book a practical teaching tool that addresses the continuing challenges of reforming the education and training of healthcare providers to deliver care that is safe and of high quality.

We are indebted to those who have helped us understand how and why to tell these stories—Tracy Granzyk, Martha Hayward, and Alide Chase, among others. The coordination and integration of the 30 contributing authors from around the world was a tremendous undertaking. We were privileged to work with talented and knowledgeable colleagues from around the globe. Above all, we are profoundly grateful to our contributors, who generously and repeatedly agreed to revise chapters, and were willing to dig deeply into painful memories in the hope that their hard-learned lessons could benefit others.

The production of this book required a team effort at all levels and in multiple locations. Antonios Lilios of the Antonios Lilios Media Group was an indispensable partner in interviewing patients, family members, and healthcare professionals. Carolyn Oliver from the Cautious Patient Foundation, Gunnar Ohlen from the Karolinska Institute, and Maureen Bisognano from the Institute of Healthcare Improvement provided invaluable support that made it possible to conduct interviews. Doug Dotan, Sir Brian Jarman, Blair Sadler, Debora Simmons, Tanya Lord, Linda Kenney, Ilene Corina, Mary Ellen Mannix, Laura Townsend, and John James volunteered much appreciated time, resources, and wisdom. Many other people shared stories and insights that helped shape the book, including interviewees whose stories space did not permit us to include in this volume. We are grateful to you all.

We would also like to acknowledge the assistance and guidance of the Editorial team at Jones & Bartlett Learning. Mike Brown, Chloe Falivene, and Lindsey Mawhiney patiently walked us through the publishing process. Our immediate and extended family members—LaBarre Blackman, Eliza Blackman, Helen Haskell Sr., David and Arlene Johnson, Harold and Frances Barach, Harrison Mohr, Tore Barach, and Elijah Barach—generously and patiently adjusted their schedules and their lives to accommodate and support this project.

And finally, we acknowledge those who have suffered due to medical harm. This book is part of our commitment and covenant to patients and their families, a compact that is possible and necessary to learn from their experiences to improve health care.

Julie K. Johnson   **Helen W. Haskell**   **Paul R. Barach**
December 2014

Robert Englander, MD, MPH

Quality and patient safety in health care have been on the forefront of the public's mind since the publication of the Institute of Medicine's seminal report *To Err Is Human* in 2000. The literature has emphasized the importance of revamping *systems and processes* to try to address the gaps in safety and quality that remain so pervasive and have eroded the public's trust. Of equal importance to the future of healthcare improvement and patient and population outcomes are the *healthcare professionals* who make up our systems of care.

Case Studies in Patient Safety: Foundations for Core Competencies invites us into the world of patients through their stories, their losses, and their suffering. It helps remind us that as healthcare professionals we devote our careers to serve patients and we need to rethink how we move from a clinician-centered to a patient- and family-centered system of care.

To be able to make this shift, we have focused over the past decade on the key desired competencies for health professionals generally and physicians specifically through their formation in education, training, and practice. Understanding why we are facing the current dilemma with health professionals not always equipped to deal with the patients, populations, and systems with which they work requires some understanding of the recent history of the notion of competencies for health professions.

Paul Batalden, a formidable figure in healthcare improvement, has among his famous quotes the statement that "Every system is perfectly designed to get the results it gets." The current design of the medical education system and the implication for its "results" is worth considering. The contemporary system of medical education remains predominantly based on the work of Abraham Flexner in 1910. His report was an indictment of the existing system of his time that was proprietary, without basis in the sciences, and without quality controls of any kind. He focused on the structure and process of medical education to ensure that physicians were grounded in the basic sciences and then exposed to clinical experiences only after that foundation was laid. He called for standards both for requisite preparation for medical school and for the basic two-by-two structure of medical school (2 years of basic science and 2 years of clinical science). The structure that emerged from that report has remained the predominant framework in most medical schools in North America today. Post medical school, internship and residency training provided an opportunity to bolster one's clinical care skills through application of basic science knowledge in the context of a specialty.

It is not surprising that this emphasis on the scientific foundations of medicine, encouraged the development of premedical education requisite sciences, and the Medical College Aptitude Test (MCAT) emerged as a way of testing that scientific knowledge prior to entering medical school. The other major contributor to one's application to medical school was the college transcript, with a particular emphasis on grades in the science courses. Thus, the premium competencies for entry into medical school and the first 2 years were clearly in the domain of Medical Knowledge. Patient Care competencies then took a prominent role during the clinical science years of the undergraduate medical education curriculum and residency training. And so it remained for the better part of a century. The medical education system was perfectly designed to attract individuals who were academically superior or who at least learned to do well on standardized tests, particularly in the sciences. They would then be expected to develop excellence in patient care skills through the clinical portions of education and training. The "results" of this system of education and training are extremely knowledgeable diagnosticians who are focused on the individual physician–patient dyad.

Why, then, are 100,000 patients dying unnecessarily every year in U.S. hospitals and millions more around the world? The answer seems to lie in the mismatch between the needs of the healthcare system and the output of the medical education system. Possessing competence in medical knowledge and patient care alone is no longer adequate to ensure quality care of patients and populations. In fact, the primacy of medical knowledge has probably declined to some extent with the advent of the information age. Information one did not carry in one's mind before the Internet explosion might take days, or even weeks, to find. Now that information is nearly all available at our fingertips 24 hours a day, 7 days a week.

As it began to be clear that Medical Knowledge and Patient Care competencies were necessary but not sufficient towards the end of the twentieth century, we began to take a new look at what it means to be a "good doctor." This work was spawned in large part in the United States by the Outcome Project of the Accreditation Council for Graduate Medical Education (Swing, 2007), in Canada by the CanMEDs project (Royal College of Physicians and Surgeons of Canada, 2005), and in Scotland by the Scottish Doctor initiative (Scottish Deans' Medical Curriculum Group, 2007). The overwhelming sentiment in all of these cases (and even some evidence) has emerged that possessing great medical knowledge and patient care skills is simply no longer adequate to be a good physician. For example, much data exists currently that physician empathy is correlated directly with patient outcomes (Hojat et al., 2011).

This novel book, through its portrayal of patient stories and suffering, powerfully illustrates the importance of competencies beyond the domains of Medical Knowledge for Practice and Patient Care. The authors use a list of 58 competencies in eight domains that the Association of American Medical Colleges published in a recent review of 153 competency lists that looked across disciplines, healthcare professions, countries, and the continuum of physician education and training. These competencies represented as best we could all of the physician competencies in those 153 lists (Englander et al.,

2013). The domains of competence began with those established by the ACGME Outcome Project: Medical Knowledge, Patient Care, Professionalism, Interpersonal and Communication Skills, Practice-Based Learning and Improvement, and Systems-Based Practice, and added the domains of Interprofessional Collaboration and Personal and Professional Development. The authors have identified the core competencies that are at work in the patient stories as a way to think about how to integrate competencies into classroom discussions.

Through a series of patient stories about medical harm they or loved ones experienced, this book provides compelling evidence that we are on the right track to defining the range of competencies required of the twenty-first-century physician. And yet, these stories also make it clear that we have a long way to go. One cannot help but be moved by these tragic stories of patients who have been made victims by the systems and individuals that let them down. What is striking as one reads these stories is the rarity with which Medical Knowledge or Patient Care competencies serve as the primary culprit in the error. To the contrary, perhaps the most common provider deficits gleaned across these stories are in the realms of Professionalism and Interpersonal and Communication Skills. How poignant, then, to underscore what is really important to being a good healthcare provider. These stories compel us to think about what competencies we really *need* our healthcare providers to possess to perform optimally in our healthcare system such as it is. And perhaps more importantly, if you are a medical educator, I implore you to think about the implications for your educational system. What is the optimal design for a system in which the final results are care providers competent in all the domains?

Finally, I hope you will be as grateful as I am to the patients and their family members for the courage and candor to share their stories. We know that courage begets courage and so these stories will help steer us in the right direction as we begin to imagine and develop a new system far different from the one imagined by Flexner over a century ago.

References

Englander, R., Cameron, T., Ballard, A. J., Dodge, J., Bull, J., & Aschenbrener, C. A. (2013). Toward a common taxonomy of competency domains for the health professions and competencies for physicians. *Academic Medicine, 88*(8), 1088–1094.

Flexner, A. (1910). *Medical education in the United States and Canada: A report to the Carnegie Foundation for the Advancement of Teaching.* New York: The Carnegie Foundation for the Advancement of Teaching.

Hojat, M., Louis, D. Z., Markham, F. W., Wender, R., Rabinowitz, C., & Gonnella, J. S. (2011). Physicians' empathy and clinical outcomes for diabetic patients. *Academic Medicine, 86*(3), 359–364.

Institute of Medicine (IOM). (2000). *To err is human: Building a safer health system.* Washington, D.C.: National Academy Press.

Royal College of Physicians and Surgeons of Canada. (2005). *The CanMEDS 2005 physician competency framework: Better standards. Better physicians. Better care.* In: Frank JR, ed. Ottawa, Ontario, Canada: The Royal College of Physicians and Surgeons of Canada. Available at: http://www. royalcollege.ca/portal/page/portal/rc/common/documents/ canmeds/resources/publications/framework_full_e.pdf.

Scottish Deans' Medical Curriculum Group (SDMCG). (2007). Learning outcomes for the medical undergraduate in Scotland: A foundation for competent and reflective practitioners. Available at: http://www. scottishdoctor.org/resources/scottishdoctor3.doc.

Swing, S. R. (2007). The ACGME outcome project: Retrospective and prospective. *Medical Teacher, 29*(7), 648–654.

Learning from Patient Stories

Julie K. Johnson, Helen W. Haskell, and Paul R. Barach

Patient safety and patient-centered quality care have emerged as key drivers across the world for healthcare reform. Although there has never been more awareness and resources devoted to overall system improvement, care experience, quality, and safety, enormous opportunities remain to achieve savings, reduce risks, and improve performance. Current approaches are not producing the pace, breadth, or magnitude of improvement that patients demand and providers expect. Patients still experience needless harm. Patients and their family members struggle to have their voices heard. Proscriptive rules, guidelines, and checklists are helping to raise awareness and prevent some harm, but these efforts fall short of providing an ultrasafe and reliable system that engages providers and empowers patients. A new system is needed—one that is centered around the needs and desires of patients and their clinical microsystems, and renders clinical care processes more predictable, effective, efficient, and humane.

One does not have to look very far to find evidence of the devastating effects of medical errors on patients and their families. All too often what is seen in the aftermath of an adverse event is a sensationalized story. The story illustrates that sometimes things can go horribly wrong and that the people who are there to help are part of a system that fails to protect the patient from more harm. This message produces fear and anger instead of inducing humility and creating an informed path forward. The stories pull at the heartstrings but fail to spur reflection, clinician engagement, and action for change. Furthermore, the stories fail to create a clear mandate for action.

We have been troubled by the repetitive nature of the errors and the tragic outcomes that emerge from the stories and the lack of systematic learning about preventing future events. In response, we set out to collect a set of stories that will help patients, their families, and their providers learn how medical errors and system failures lead to patient harm. The idea for the book is based on the story of Lewis Blackman, a 15-year-old boy who died from complications following elective surgery. We published a case study on Lewis's experience (Johnson et al., 2012), and we were delighted to discover that the case study approach was well received and a powerful way to share Lewis's story as well as an effective method to teach about system failures, medical error, and harm prevention. When using the case as a teaching tool, we would first share the story from the family's perspective, provide a brief analysis of the events, and then invite learners to reflect on and discuss what could be learned from the event. We were asked if we had other stories to share about patient harm from medical error, and that is how this book came to life.

Our aim is to present the stories as told from the firsthand perspective of the patient and family. This presented us with a challenge in developing the case studies because, like a Rashomon, there are multiple perspectives to each story. We chose to tell the story from the unique perspective of the patient. We acknowledge that this may present a limited and incomplete retelling of the "full facts" as they unfolded. The stories we present are the patients' perceptions and their reality, regardless of whether all the details can be supported by the evidence at hand. In the end, we agreed that we wanted to ensure that the patient's voice would be heard, highlighting their mental model and mind-set as they experienced, witnessed, and understood the events.

The cases presented are devastating accounts of the harm and suffering experienced by the patient and their family. While developing the book, colleagues would ask us, "Why are you focusing on the bad stories when there are so many stories with good outcomes? Shouldn't we learn from those, too?" And they are right. Our healthcare systems, across the world, have shining examples of how caregivers can heal and provide life-sustaining interventions, most of the time. However, we believe that for healthcare systems to become reliably better, that is, to deliver safe and high quality care all the time, we need to enlist patients, families, and their stories. For us, this is, as Kierkegaard said, about "meeting people where they are." To do that, we need to allow patients and families to share their experiences and stories in their own voices, and to accept that their experiences have profound lessons for us all.

The book presents a challenge on how to think differently about how best to emotionally and intellectually engage patients and healthcare providers in healthcare transformation, which is the core work of this generation of caring professionals. We welcome your feedback about how you use these cases, as well as your suggestions and ideas for improvement.

Reference

Johnson, J., Haskell, H., & Barach, P. (2012). The Lewis Blackman Hospital Patient Safety Act: It's hard to kill a healthy 15-year-old. In: McLaughlin, C., Johnson, J., & Sollecito, W. (eds.), *Implementing continuous quality improvement in health care: A global casebook*. Sudbury, MA: Jones & Bartlett Learning.

Setting the Stage for Case Studies in Patient Safety: Foundations for Core Competencies

Julie K. Johnson, Paul R. Barach, and Helen W. Haskell

"People must always come before numbers. It is the individual experiences that lie behind statistics and benchmarks and action plans that really matter, and that is what must never be forgotten when policies are being made and implemented."

—Robert Francis (2010)

Francis, R. (2010). *Return to an Address of the Honourable the House of Commons dated 24 February 2010: Independent Inquiry into care provided by Mid Staffordshire NHS Foundation Trust January 2005–March 2009*. London: Stationery Office.

Donald Schön speaks of the challenges in implementing meaningful change as moving from "The ivory tower to the swampy lowland" (Schön, 1983). We take this to mean that if health care as an industry aims to provide patient care that is safe and of high quality and value, we must move from academic theory and rhetoric to implementation strategies that are grounded in the chaotic day-to-day challenges of making health care safer. Stories of patient experiences, especially those that highlight the gaps, inconsistencies, and errors in the care-giving process can offer the bridge from theory to implementing improvement.

They contribute to the ever growing number of providers who are burnt out, disengaged and eager to leave health care. Two separate, but closely related, forces drive this book—the need to improve the quality, safety, and value of health care for patients, and, the need to improve education, training, and joy of healthcare professionals. When designing strategies to improve patient safety and health professionals' education, patients and their families cannot be overlooked. The stories of patient harm as told from the perspectives of patients and their families are the bridge between theory and action for improving education and practice.

We believe in the role and power of stories to effect change. Novelist Robert Moss likes to quote the Australian Aborigines as saying that the big stories—the stories worth telling and retelling, the ones in which you may find the meaning of your life—are forever stalking the right teller, sniffing and tracking like predators hunting their prey (Moss, 1998). The stories in this book have haunted us in this way. Our hope is that these stories will hold this sort of deep meaning for those who read and use them. On an educational plane, our goal is that the book will (1) support the use of patient stories to address multiple intercalated competencies across the health professions; (2) guide the formation of junior health professionals, as well as the continued development and life-long learning of established health professionals; (3) provide the foundation for lifelong learning focused around the patient journey; and (4) prompt dialogue among the healthcare training and delivery communities about how to more effectively use patient stories to improve and assess inter-professional core competencies.

This introduction sets the stage for *Case Studies in Patient Safety: Foundations for Core Competencies.* We start with an overview of the magnitude of the problem of medical errors and patient harm, present lack of clinician engagement as a barrier to improving quality and safety of care, and discuss how patients are at the heart of improvement work. We outline the role of systems improvement efforts and how safety science has helped reconceptualize clinical risk. Regulators, accreditors, and policy makers have been front and center in incentivizing better care by more effective incentive alignment, which leads us directly into a discussion about the formation of health professionals, including education, training, and accreditation. We present a set of core competencies for health professions and discuss the challenges educators face in teaching these competencies to individuals as well as to healthcare teams. Finally, we make the case for the unique power of patient stories to engage providers and consumers and outline how the case studies included in the book fit into the core competency framework and become a central part of all healthcare training.

The Impact of Medical Errors and Patient Harm

More than a decade has passed since the Institute of Medicine (IOM) published reports that focused national, as well as international, attention on the problem of medical errors and preventable harm to patients (IOM, 1999, 2001). The magnitude of the problem, as estimated by the IOM of as many as 98,000 deaths in U.S. hospitals per year, was initially hotly debated, but has since been widely accepted and replicated in other studies around the world. Although some questioned the validity of these numbers, a careful review suggests that these numbers are conservative estimates. Any estimate of an error rate is inexact, due to limitations of:

- Methods of data collection, analysis, and interpretation
- Unknown levels of underreporting (Pietro, Shyavitz, Smith, & Auerbach, 2000)
- Difficulty of retrospective analysis (Hayward & Hofer, 2001; McNutt, Abrams, & Arons, 2002)

The problem of medical errors leading to patient harm is not unique to the U.S. healthcare system. Across the world, people seeking care in hospitals are harmed 9.2% of the time, with death occurring in 7.4% of these events (de Vries et al., 2008). Furthermore, it is estimated that 43.5% of these harm events are preventable. A recent study that extrapolated the results of four studies that used a global trigger tool to identify medical error estimated that the number of patients harmed in the United States may be much higher—between 210,000 and 440,000 patient deaths each year (James, 2013). Based on statistics from the Centers for Disease Control (CDC) about the leading causes of death in the United States, these updated estimates would make medical errors the third leading cause of death, following heart disease and cancer (CDC, 2013). These estimates are reflected in studies from several countries (Davis, Stremikis, Schoen, & Squires, 2014).

The potential for patient harm does not stop at the hospital doors. It has been reported that nearly 1 in 5 patients suffers adverse events fairly soon after coming home from the hospital (Traynor, 2003). In one study, 76 of 400 consecutively discharged patients suffered a total of 78 adverse events within 5 weeks after being discharged home from the hospital. Twenty-three of the adverse events were deemed to be preventable, and 24 were classified as ameliorable (i.e., of a severity that could have been greatly reduced by altering procedures for patient care).

The evidence base supporting strategies to improve patient safety is now stronger than ever before (Shekelle et al., 2013; Wachter, Pronovost, & Shekelle, 2013). A body of evidence has emerged that highlights the types of errors that frequently occur and has identified medical error as a major public health problem that cannot be ignored. Progress has been made on multiple fronts during the past several decades. Patient safety and patient-centered care have become key drivers in healthcare reform. Clinicians, researchers, and policy makers have worked to improve the safety of patient care. Regulators, accreditors, and payers incentivize healthcare organizations to improve patient safety and reduce preventable adverse events by adopting evidence-based patient safety practices that reduce preventable adverse events.

Yet, despite large investments in effort and financial resources, we continue to see the effects of solutions that do not address the underlying systems of care and fail to recognize the context-dependent nature of clinical improvement (Phelps & Barach, 2014). Patients often struggle to have their voices heard. Processes of care are not as efficient as they could be, and costs continue to rise at alarming rates, while quality and safety issues remain.

Early efforts at improving safety were somewhat naïve. According to Wachter and colleagues (2013), there were beliefs that "adopting some techniques drawn from aviation and other 'safe industries,' building strong information technology systems, and improving patient safety culture" would result in safer systems of care and improved patient safety. These efforts often paid scant attention to the underlying culture and misaligned financial and political incentives. In reality, safer patient care requires ongoing, systematic efforts guided by strong, value-based, and courageous leadership that is willing to be truthful to clinicians and patients about the challenges ahead. Building reliability into healthcare operations can only occur with a culture of transparency and reflection designed with the patient and the clinical microsystems at the frontlines of care.

Lack of Clinician Engagement as a Barrier to Improving Quality and Safety of Care

Misalignment of financial incentives, lack of clear transparent accountability, and limited clinician engagement remain the biggest obstacles in addressing the growing implementation gap in providing cost-effective, high-quality care. Physician discontent and cynicism and the growing numbers of burnt-out clinicians all point to a serious gap in trust and lack of engagement in clinical improvement (Jorm, 2012). Engaging clinicians and creating authentic partnerships are key to facilitation of clinician adoption of new care models and to reigniting the passion and loyalty of healthcare providers to their avocation.

Effective improvement of care will require meaningful efforts to address the engagement gap with clinicians in large part because new care models require doctors to significantly change their behavior. Trust-building steps in which clinicians can see and understand the value and effort in implementing improvement strategies are key. Lencioni (2002) posits that teams fail because they fall prey to five dysfunctions that undermine their cohesiveness and reliability:

1. Absence of trust
2. Fear of conflict
3. Lack of commitment
4. Avoidance of accountability
5. Inattention to results

Members of effective cohesive teams learn to trust one another, but only if they are able to engage and challenge each other in a respectful manner around ideas, commit to decisions and plans of action, hold one another accountable for delivering against those plans, and focus on the achievement of collective results.

Patients at the Heart of Improvement

Patient-centered care has been defined as care that is respectful of, and responsive to, individual patient preferences, needs, and values and ensures that patient values guide all clinical decisions (IOM, 2001).

The current fragmentation of healthcare services makes effective application of a patient-centered model of quality improvement difficult, if not impossible. Care that is truly patient centered can only be achieved with active patient engagement at every level of care design and implementation. Patients who feel respected, attended to, and in full partnership of their care are more compliant with their medications and medical appointments, feel better about their care, and have better overall health (Blue Shield of California, 2012).

At the most basic, patient-centered care involves a reconceptualization of the patient from the passive object of medical intervention to an active "consumer" or "user" of health services who *coproduces and "owns" his or her own health.* Reframing of patient care is needed from a task-oriented, practitioner-centered model to a systems-based, patient-centered model that looks to the actual relationships within the sociotechnical microsystems in which care is actually delivered (Barach & Johnson, 2006). This must also include a commitment to full disclosure when things go awry, setting up peer support programs for clinicians who have harmed patients, and long-term support for patients, families, and providers who are involved in adverse care (Australian Commission on Safety and Quality in Healthcare, 2011).

Safety Science and Systems Improvement

There has been an important reconceptualization of clinical risk through the emphasis on how upstream "latent factors" enable, condition, or exacerbate the potential for "active errors" and patient harm. Decades of work within and outside health care point to system flaws that conspire and set good people up to fail. Understanding the characteristics of a safe, resilient, and high-performing system requires research to optimize the dynamic relationships between people, tasks, and their organizational and physical environments (Mohr & Batalden, 2006). The sociotechnical approach suggests that adverse incidents can be examined from both an organizational perspective that incorporates both the concept of latent conditions and the cascading nature of human error, commencing with management decisions and actions (or inactions). Organizational resilience is found in the responsiveness of care delivery teams to an emerging hazard. Some teams are more resilient than others and are able to recover from failed decisions and processes. That is, they are able to recover from errors reliably and reduce future patient harm, whereas others contribute to patient harm, do not learn from their errors, and repeat them (Hollangel, Woods, & Leveson, 2006).

People often find ways of getting around processes that seem to be unnecessary or that impede the workflow. This is known as *normalization of deviance*. By a deviant organizational behavior, we are referring to "an event, activity or circumstance, occurring in and/or produced by a formal organization that deviates from both formal design goals and normative standards or expectations, either in the fact of its occurrence or in its consequences" (Vaughn, 1999). Once a community normalizes a deviant organizational practice, it is no longer viewed as an aberrant act that elicits an exceptional response; instead, it becomes a routine activity that is commonly anticipated and frequently used (Vaughan, 1996).

A permissive ethical climate, an emphasis on financial goals at all costs, and an opportunity to act amorally or immorally all contribute to managerial decisions to initiate deviance (Earle et al., 2010). This accumulated acceptance of cutting corners or making workarounds over time poses a great danger to health care. Similar findings have been described in investigations into major episodes of clinical failure, suggesting that health systems are failing to heed the lessons of history (Dyer, 2001; Queensland Health Systems Review, 2005).

Incentivizing Better Care: Regulators, Accreditors, and Policy Makers

Major changes are needed in the design and delivery of effective healthcare systems. Given the pressures to deliver better value, the systems that will thrive will focus on quality of care (including cost-efficiency) through innovative healthcare delivery that results from the alignment of incentives with payers, patients, and other participants in the healthcare equation. Jim Collins (2001), in his seminal book *From Good to Great*, underscores the fundamental need for leaders to address misaligned incentives and encouraging employees to speak up to produce reliable outcomes.

The Joint Commission (TJC) revamped its regulatory framework focusing on clinician engagement given the ongoing data suggesting that, despite much regulatory effort, harm in healthcare systems continued to happen. In 2002, TJC established the National Patient Safety Goals (NPSGs) program to help accredited organizations address specific areas of concern with regard to patient safety and to create national benchmarks that were evidence based and that could be upheld in public.

Payers have been focusing on this misalignment and providing financial incentives to improve the quality and safety of patient care. For example, in 2008 Medicare stopped reimbursing hospitals for treating eight avoidable hospital-acquired conditions—foreign object retained after surgery, air embolism, blood incompatibility, stages III and IV pressure ulcers, in-hospital falls and trauma, catheter-associated urinary tract infection (UTI), vascular catheter–associated infection, and certain surgical site infections—as a way to discourage and penalize hospitals for poor-quality care and encourage them to eliminate avoidable complications.

Equally, around the world, the findings of the Francis Report into the failings of care at the UK Mid Staffordshire Hospital (Francis, 2010), the Special Commission into Acute Care Services in New South Wales Public Hospitals (Garling Inquiry) (Garling, 2008), and the cover-up by the Clinical Quality Commission (CQC) of the University Hospitals of Morecambe Bay NHS Trust (Care Quality Commission, 2013) highlight the problems with lax regulatory oversight (Vaughan, 1999). These inquiries found that during the periods under investigation many staff, patients, and managers had raised concerns about the standard of care provided to patients. The tragedy was that they were ignored and the concerns were covered up. Senior managers seemed more concerned about protecting their reputation and their next job than about the lives of patients in the systems under their oversight (Care Quality Commission, 2013). Finally, and perhaps of most concern, these public reports documented a widespread culture of denial, a lack of attentiveness to patient concerns, and pervasive normalized deviance (Vaughan, 1999).

Implications for Training and Education

The IOM (1999) recommended a focus on the initial and continuing education and training of healthcare professionals in order to have the greatest impact. The IOM recommended that healthcare organizations make patient safety a priority by establishing patient safety programs that would "establish interdisciplinary team training programs, that incorporate proven methods for team management" (p. 135). The IOM also recommended that standards and expectations for healthcare organizations and professionals place a greater emphasis on team-based patient safety. The IOM proposed that such standards should mandate periodic recertification and relicensing of doctors, nurses, and other key providers. Recertification would focus both on provider competence and on knowledge of patient safety practices, such as functioning effectively in an interdisciplinary healthcare team.

At the heart of efforts to improve patient safety, we need an approach to healthcare training that produces professionals who not only demonstrate competence in clinical skills, but who are also accountable to a core set of competencies, with competency defined as "an observable and measureable ability, integrating multiple components such as knowledge, skills, values, and attitudes" (Englander et al., 2013). The gap between training of healthcare professionals and meeting patient needs remains wide. We need reliable and valid measures to diagnose learning deficiencies, provide accurate feedback, and where appropriate, select appropriate strategies for remediation.

Core Competencies for Health Professions Education

Education has shifted toward competency-based education across the health professions with varied competency frameworks emerging from different countries. For example, frameworks for physician competencies have been developed in different countries—these include the Outcome Project of the Accreditation

Council for Graduate Medical Education (ACGME) (Swing, 2007) and American Board of Medical Specialties (ABMS) in the United States, the CanMEDS Framework of the Royal College of Physicians and Surgeons of Canada (Curriculum & Group, 2007), the Scottish Doctor Project in Scotland (Curriculum & Group, 2007), and the Framework for Undergraduate Medical Education in the Netherlands (Laan, Leunissen, & Van Herwaarden, 2010). Some health professions, such as nursing, have used competency frameworks for decades, although integration of core competencies into health professions education can be slow. Although different disciplines recognize the value of competency-based education, there has not been a common set of competencies for health professionals. Englander and colleagues reviewed 153 health professions' competency lists, to identify a robust list of competency domains, published as of June 2012 that could accommodate all healthcare professions. **Table FM-1** summarizes the eight competency domains. The full set (58 competencies) is included in the appendix. The Association of American Medical Colleges (AAMC) has put forth the list as a recommended common taxonomy of competencies for research and educators within medicine and other health professions (Englander et al., 2013).

These competency domains have implications for health professional education, training, and accreditation. Some of the domains represent areas that have been taught and assessed as part of the rich tradition of health professions education, for example, Patient Care and Knowledge for Practice. Other domains, such as Systems-Based Practice and Practice-Based Learning and Improvement, are more challenging for educators to assess, and they continue to struggle with teaching these competencies to individuals as well as to healthcare teams functioning within a clinical microsystem. The competencies have improved our understanding in describing a framework of professionalism, but they challenge educators especially in regards to education, assessment readiness to practice.

Table FM-1 Competency Domains

Competency Domain	Definition of Competence
Patient Care	Provide patient-centered care that is compassionate, appropriate, and effective for the treatment of health problems and the promotion of health.
Knowledge for Practice	Demonstrate knowledge of established and evolving biomedical, clinical, epidemiological, and social-behavioral sciences, as well as the application of this knowledge to patient care.
Practice-Based Learning and Improvement	Demonstrate the ability to investigate and evaluate one's care of patients, to appraise and assimilate scientific evidence, and to continuously improve patient care based on constant self-evaluation and lifelong learning.
Interpersonal and Communication Skills	Demonstrate interpersonal and communication skills that result in the effective exchange of information and collaboration with patients, their families, and health professionals.
Professionalism	Demonstrate a commitment to carrying out professional responsibilities and an adherence to ethical principles.
Systems-Based Practice	Demonstrate an awareness of and responsiveness to the larger context and system of health care, as well as the ability to call effectively on other resources in the system to provide optimal health care.
Interprofessional Collaboration	Demonstrate the ability to engage in an interprofessional team in a manner that optimizes safe, effective patient- and population-centered care.
Personal and Professional Development	Demonstrate the qualities required to sustain lifelong personal and professional growth.

Englander, R. et al. 2013. Toward a Common Taxonomy of Competency Domains for the Health Professions and Competencies for Physicians. *Acad Med, 88,* 1088-1094.

The Power of the Patient Story in Teaching Core Competencies

Patient stories capture the rich complexity and dynamic progression of the patient journey and offer a rare opportunity for providers and teachers to explore the competency domains beyond direct patient care and discipline-specific knowledge. This text, *Case Studies in Patient Safety: Foundations for Core Competencies*, makes an effort to systematize the telling and recording of stories of patient harm, the learning from these stories, and strategies for how we apply them in progressing a competency-based framework. The patient stories offer a way to integrate and teach health professional core competencies in a manner that is both relevant and engaging for clinicians. Using the core competencies as a lens and a guide for thinking about the cases, the competencies can support and encourage high-value, patient-centered care for patients and their families. Our focus on complex real-world patient cases ensures that patients and their experiences are always at the center of all educational efforts. In real life, patient care does not come neatly compartmentalized into discrete categories. The biggest challenge educators face in actuating the competencies for healthcare professionals is that the individual competencies are isolated and difficult to assess in the reductionist approach that is commonplace in healthcare delivery systems.

The stories we have collected are contextualized and grounded within the clinical microsystem, or multiple microsystems, which allow a holistic integration of the core competencies, while respecting the patient journey. The stories address and bring together the medical knowledge in the cases with the social, sociological, and relational aspects of the patient–provider interaction. The book is organized into eight sections, each representing a core competency. Each section starts with a brief overview of the competency and a description of the case studies that are included in the section. Each case is presented in a consistent format, an editors' note that provides the context, specific learning objectives for the case, the story as told from the patient/family perspective, and a case discussion written by the editors to prompt thinking about some of the relevant patient safety issues. The case ends with questions for classroom discussion.

The allocation of cases to a particular competency is based on how well the case describes elements of that competency. Many of the cases relate to and touch upon multiple competencies. For example, in Case 1, Lewis Blackman's death in the hospital following surgery, was allocated to the section on Patient Care, but it is also relevant and requires Knowledge for Practice, Professionalism, and Interpersonal and Communication Skills. The final section in this book is Personal and Professional Development. This book of case studies provides a vehicle for Personal and Professional Development, where health professionals "demonstrate the qualities required to sustain lifelong personal and professional growth."

References

Australian Commission on Safety and Quality in Healthcare. (2011). *Patient-centred care: Improving safety and quality through partnerships with patients and consumers*. Sydney: Author.

Barach, P., & Johnson, J. (2006). Understanding the complexity of redesigning care around the clinical microsystem. *Quality & Safety in Health Care, 15*(Suppl 1), i10–i16.

Blue Shield of California. (2012). *Empowerment and engagement among low-income Californians: Enhancing patient-centered care*. San Francisco: Author.

Care Quality Commission. (2013). Project Ambrose.

Centers for Disease Control and Prevention (CDC). (2013). Leading causes of death. Available at: http://www.cdc.gov/nchs/fastats/lcod.htm.

Collins, J. (2001). *Good to great: Why some companies make the leap and others don't*. New York: Harper Collins.

Curriculum & Group. (2007). *Learning outcomes for the medical undergraduate in Scotland: A foundation for competent and reflective practitioners* (3rd ed.). Dundee, Scotland: AMEE Office.

Davis, K., Stremikis, K., Schoen, C., & Squires D. *Mirror, Mirror on the Wall, 2014 Update: How the U.S. Health Care System Compares Internationally*, The Commonwealth Fund, June 2014.

De Vries, E., Ramrattan, M., Smorenburg, S., Gouma, D., & Boermeester, M. (2008). The incidence and nature of in-hospital adverse events: A systematic review. *Quality and Safety in Health Care, 17,* 216–223.

Dyer, C. (2001). Bristol inquiry condemns hospital's "club culture." BMJ, 323, 181.

Earle, J., Spicer, A., & Peter K. S. (April 2010). The normalization of deviant organizational practices: Wage arrears in Russia, 1992-1998. *Academy of Management Journal. 53*:2, 218–237.

Englander, R., Cameron, T., Ballard, A. J., Dodge, J., Bull, J., & Aschenbrener, C. A. (2013). Toward a common taxonomy of competency domains for the health professions and competencies for physicians. *Academic Medicine, 88,* 1088–1094.

Francis, R. (2010). *Independent inquiry into care provided by Mid Staffordshire NHS Foundation Trust.* London: The Stationery Office.

Garling, P. (2008). *Final Report of the Special Commission of Inquiry: Acute care in NSW public hospitals.* New South Wales, Australia, State of NSW.

Hayward, R. A., & Hofer, T. P. (2001). Estimating hospital deaths due to medical errors: Preventability is in the eye of the reviewer. *JAMA, 286,* 415–420.

Hollangel, E., Woods, D., & Leveson, N. (eds.). (2006). *Resilience engineering: Concepts and precepts.* Aldershot, England: Ashgate.

Institute of Medicine. (1999). *To err is human: Building a safer health system.* Washington, D.C.: National Academy Press.

Institute of Medicine. (2001). *Crossing the quality chasm: A new health system for the 21st century.* Washington, D.C.: National Academy Press.

James, J. (2013). A new, evidence-based estimate of patient harms associated with hospital care. *Journal of Patient Safety, 9,* 122–128.

Jorm, C. (2012). Reconstructing medical practice: Engagement, professionalism and critical relationships in health care. Surrey, UK: Gower.

Laan, R. F., Leunissen, R. R., & Van Herwaarden, C. L. (2010). The 2009 framework for undergraduate medical education in the Netherlands. *German Journal for Medical Education* (*GMS Z Med Ausbild*), 27, Doc35.

Lencioni, P. (2002). *The five dysfunctions of a team.* San Francisco: Jossey-Bass.

Moss, R. (1998). Dreamgates: An explorer's guide to the worlds of soul, imagination, and life beyond death. New York: Three Rivers Press.

McNutt, R. A., Abrams, R., & Arons, D. C. (2002). Patient safety efforts should focus on medical errors. *JAMA, 287,* 1997–2001.

Mohr, J., & Batalden, P. (2006). Integrating approaches to health professional development with approaches to improving patient care. In: McLaughlin, C., & Kaluzny, A. (eds.), *Continuous quality improvement in health care: Theory, implementations, and applications* (3rd ed.). Boston: Jones & Bartlett.

Phelps, G., & Barach, P. (2014). Why the safety and quality movement has been slow to improve care? *International Journal of Clinical Practice, 68*(8), 932–935.

Pietro, D. A., Shyavitz, L. J., Smith, R. A., & Auerbach, B. S. (2000). Detecting and reporting medical errors: Why the dilemma? *BMJ, 320,* 794–796.

Queensland Health Systems Review. (2005).

Schön, D. (1983). *The reflective practitioner: How professionals think in action.* New York: Basic Books.

Shekelle, P. G., Pronovost, P. J., Wachter, R. M., McDonald, K. M., Schoelles, K., . . . Walshe, K. (2013). The top patient safety strategies that can be encouraged for adoption now. *Annals of Internal Medicine, 158,* 365–368.

Swing, S. R. (2007). The ACGME outcome project: Retrospective and prospective. *Medical Teacher, 29,* 648–654.

Traynor, K. (2003). Adverse events occur after hospital discharge, study finds. *American Journal of Health-System Pharmacy, 60,* 534.

Vaughan, D. (1996). *The Challenger launch decision: Risky technology, culture, and deviance at NASA.* Chicago: University of Chicago Press.

Vaughan, D. (1999). The dark side of organizations: Mistake, misconduct, and disaster. *Annual Review of Sociology, 25,* 271–305.

Wachter, R. M., Pronovost, P., & Shekelle, P. (2013). Strategies to improve patient safety: The evidence base matures. *Annals of Internal Medicine, 158,* 350–352.

Patient Care

Healthcare professionals must be able to demonstrate the provision of patient-centered care that is compassionate, appropriate, and effective for the treatment of health problems and the promotion of health. Specific competencies within the Patient Care domain are to:

- Perform medical, diagnostic, and surgical procedures considered essential for the area of practice.
- Gather essential and accurate information about patients and their conditions through history-taking, physical examination, and the use of laboratory data, imaging, and other tests.
- Organize and prioritize responsibilities to provide care that is safe, effective, and efficient.
- Interpret laboratory data, imaging studies, and other tests required for the area of practice.
- Make informed decisions about diagnostic and therapeutic interventions based on patient information and preferences, up-to-date scientific evidence, and clinical judgment.
- Develop and carry out patient management plans.
- Counsel and educate patients and their families and empower them to participate in their care and enable shared decision making.

- Provide appropriate referral of patients, including ensuring continuity of care throughout transitions between providers or settings, and following up on patient progress and outcomes.
- Provide healthcare services to patients, families, and communities aimed at preventing health problems and maintaining health.
- Provide appropriate role modeling.
- Perform supervisory responsibilities commensurate with one's roles, abilities, and qualifications.

The four cases presented in Section 1 represent a range of events, types of patients, and care settings that illustrate and demonstrate key elements of the Patient Care domain. The cases are complex and include elements of other competency domains as well. As you read the cases, think about the other competencies that are relevant. (Refer to the full list of competencies in the appendix.)

The first case relates to Lewis Blackman's postoperative death following an elective surgery at an academic medical center hospital in the United States. Lewis was 15 years old when he underwent surgery for a congenital abnormality, pectus excavatum. Case 1, "It's Hard to Kill a Healthy 15-Year-Old," was the impetus for this book of case studies.

Case 2, "Routine Appendectomy," is set in Perth, Australia. Sandra Pintabona, a nurse, shares the tragic story of her husband's surgery and postoperative complications. Now, more than a decade later, John has never fully recovered from these events. Sandra Pintabona writes about her challenges as a senior healthcare professional in navigating the healthcare system to get the best care for her husband.

Julie Bailey wrote Case 3, "The Origins of the Mid Staffordshire Inquiry into the National Health Service," about her mother's death at the Mid Staffordshire Hospital in the United Kingdom. Bella Bailey was admitted to the hospital with a hiatal hernia. Julie's observation of the substandard care of her mother and other inpatients ultimately led to the Mid Staffordshire Inquiry—the largest inquiry of its kind, commissioned in 2010 to examine the care provided by the UK's National Health Service (NHS).

The final case in this section, Case 4, is about the death of James Mannix in the United States. In the summer of 2001, Mary Ellen and Michael Mannix learned from a prenatal echocardiogram that their fourth child, James, had a high chance of being born with a heart defect. In Case 4, "Consent and Disclosure in Pediatric Heart Surgery," Mary Ellen Mannix writes about James's death just days after birth due to a series of medical errors and system failures.

It's Hard to Kill a Healthy 15-Year-Old

The Story of Lewis Blackman (United States)

Helen Haskell, Julie Johnson, and Paul Barach

Editors' Note

Lewis Blackman was born with pectus excavatum, which literally means "hollowed chest." It is a congenital abnormality of the anterior wall of the chest that results in abnormal growth of the sternum and the adjoining sections of ribs. Whereas mild cases may only result in a sunken appearance of the chest, more severe cases may be associated with impaired cardiac and respiratory function (Crump, 1992; Shamberger, 1996). Many people with pectus excavatum also suffer from negative body image and self-esteem (Medline, 2007), and patients may seek surgical correction for either physical or psychological reasons. In the United States, pectus excavatum is thought to occur in about 1 in 300 to 400 white male births, with a male-to-female ratio of approximately 5:1. Although data are limited, there is reason to believe that the international incidence is approximately the same in most populations. The defect appears to be rare in persons of African descent (Jaroszewski et al., 2010).

Lewis underwent surgery for his pectus condition at age 15. He died 4 days later, without ever having left the hospital. Helen Haskell, Lewis's mother, tells the story of the events surrounding her son's surgery and death. Since Lewis's death, Helen has worked on patient safety issues in the United States and internationally by organizing parents and medical error victims into a mutual support group, Mothers Against Medical Error.

LEARNING OBJECTIVES

After completing this case study, you will be able to:

1. Outline the elements of an effective informed consent process.
2. Hypothesize the effect of professional hierarchy on communication patterns, patient care, and patient safety.
3. Evaluate the causes of failure to recognize and act upon acute deterioration in patients.
4. Discuss the elements of the Lewis Blackman Patient Safety Act as an example of the patient perspective on communication problems in hospitals.

The Decision to Operate

Taking Lewis for the pectus surgery was not an easy decision. His pectus defect, although noticeable, was relatively mild and did not cause any obvious problems. An easygoing boy, Lewis was an avid soccer player who had no evident impairment in stamina, and he was not particularly self-conscious about the concavity in his chest. He was also a high-achieving ninth-grader with a busy schedule from which he was not eager to take time out. We had never considered seeking surgical correction until we saw a newspaper article promoting a new, minimally invasive surgery that was supposed to be safer and quicker than the older method of opening the chest and remodeling the ribs and cartilage. We discussed the options with our family physician and made an appointment with a surgeon. The evidence presented by the surgeon was limited, but we decided to go ahead with the minimally invasive surgery because we were told that the procedure would become more difficult as Lewis got older. The operation was to be performed at a leading academic medical center several hours from our home. The entire family—Lewis, his younger sister, my husband, and I—spent the night in a hotel and arrived at the hospital on a Thursday morning for the surgery.

At the Hospital

Upon arrival at the hospital, we were surrounded by activity as nurses and residents took Lewis's vital signs, filled out forms, and asked us to sign documents. One of the documents, not particularly emphasized, was a one-paragraph consent form for the surgery. By 7:00 a.m., Lewis had been whisked away to surgery. When the surgeon came out later, he told us the operation had gone well, but it took longer than we expected—2 and a half hours instead of the anticipated 45 minutes. (**Figure 1-1** uses process mapping to summarize the tragic series of events that transpired over the next 4 days leading to Lewis's death.)

The first sign we had of a potential problem occurred in the recovery room, when the nurse told us that Lewis was producing abnormally low amounts of urine. In spite of this, he was prescribed a standard 5-day adult dose of the intravenous nonsteroidal anti-inflammatory (NSAID) painkiller ketorolac (trade name: Toradol). This medication should be used with caution in patients with low fluid output and was not approved for use in children younger than 16. Nevertheless, Lewis's condition appeared to be generally stable for the first 3 days in the hospital. But on Sunday, the morning of the fourth postoperative day, half an hour after a ketorolac injection Lewis was suddenly overcome by severe pain in the upper abdomen. Nurses and a medical intern were initially concerned, but then assured us that he was suffering from postoperative constipation that would resolve if he got out of bed and began moving around. However, his condition continued to worsen, and his vital signs began to deteriorate in an alarming way. Here is a quote from my journal describing what happened later that day:

It is now afternoon. Lewis's bowels and urinary system are still not functioning. His belly is hard and distended and he is extremely pale, with a subnormal temperature and a constant cold sweat. His eyes are sunken and surrounded by huge black circles. Lewis is exhausted and in agony. His pain is now radiating to the shoulder. He is also nauseated and often burps, a new symptom. He still tries not to throw up, because he has been told the fruit juice he has drunk will help revitalize his digestive system.

We call the nurse a number of times. She seems to be convinced that Lewis is simply lazy and not walking enough to dissipate his "gas pain." Sometimes no

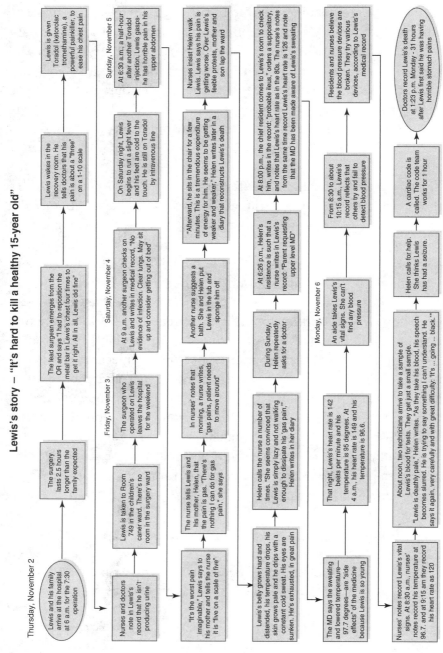

Lewis's story — "It's hard to kill a healthy 15-year old"

Thursday, November 2

Lewis and his family arrive at the hospital at 6 a.m. for the 7:30 operation

The surgery lasts 2.5 hours longer than the family expected

The lead surgeon emerges from the OR and says "I had to reposition the metal bar in Lewis's chest four times to get it right. All in all, Lewis did fine"

Lewis wakes in the recovery room. He tells doctors that his pain is about a "three" on a 1-10 scale

Lewis is given Toradol (ketorolac tromethamine), a powerful painkiller, to ease his chest pain

Sunday, November 5

At 6:30 a.m., a half-hour after another Toradol injection, Lewis gasps—he has horrible pain in his upper abdomen

Nurses insist Helen walk Lewis. Lewis says his pain is getting worse. Over Lewis's feeble protests, mother and son lap the ward

Friday, November 3

Nurses and doctors note in Lewis's record that he isn't producing urine

Lewis is taken to Room 749 in the children's caner ward. There's no room in the surgery ward

The surgeon who operated on Lewis leaves the hospital for the weekend

Saturday, November 4

At 9 a.m. another surgeon checks on Lewis and writes in medical record, "No evidence of infection. Clear lungs. May sit up and consider getting out of bed"

On Saturday night, Lewis begins to run a slight fever and his feet are cold to the touch. He is still on Toradol by intravenous line

"Afterward, he sits in the chair for a few minutes. This is a tremendous expenditure of energy for him. He seems to be getting weaker and weaker," Helen writes later in a diary that reconstructs Lewis's death

At 8:00 p.m., the chief resident comes to Lewis's room to check him, writes in the record: "probable ileus," orders a suppository, and notes that Lewis's heart rate is in the 80s. The nurse's notes from the same time record Lewis's heart rate is 126 and note that the MD has been made aware of Lewis's sweating

Residents and nurses believe the blood pressure devices are broken. They try various devices, according to Lewis's medical record

The nurse tells Lewis and his mother, Helen, that the pain is gas. "There's nothing I can do for gas pain," she says

In nurses' notes that morning, a nurse writes, "gas pains, patient needs to move around"

Another nurse suggests a bath. She and Helen put Lewis in the tub and sponge him off

During Sunday, Helen repeatedly asks for a doctor

At 6:26 p.m., Helen's insistence is such that a nurse writes in Lewis's record: "Parent requesting upper level MD"

From 8:30 to about 10:15 a.m., Lewis's record reflects that others try and fail to detect blood pressure

Doctors record Lewis's death at 1:23 p.m. Monday - 31 hours after Lewis first said he was having horrible stomach pains

"It's the worst pain imaginable," Lewis says to his mother even—tells the nurse it is "five on a scale of five"

Helen calls the nurse a number of times. "She seems convinced that Lewis is simply lazy and not walking enough to dissipate his 'gas pain,'" Helen writes in her diary

Monday, November 6

An aide takes Lewis's vital signs. She can't find any blood pressure

Helen calls for help. She thinks Lewis has had a seizure.

A cardiac code is called. The code team works for 1 hour

Lewis's belly grows hard and distended, his temperature drops, his skin grows pale and he drips with a constant cold sweat. His eyes are sunken. He's exhausted, in great pain

That night, Lewis's heart rate is 142 beats per minute and his temperature is 95 degrees. At 4 a.m., his heart rate is 149 and his temperature is 96.6.

About noon, two technicians arrive to take a sample of Lewis's blood for tests. They get just a small sample. "Lewis is deathly pale," Helen writes. "As they take his blood, his speech becomes slurred. He is trying to say something I can't understand. He says it again, very carefully and with great difficulty: 'It's ... going ... black. '"

The MD says the sweating and lowered temperature—97.7 degrees—are "side effects" of the medicine because Lewis is so young

Nurses' notes record Lewis's vital signs. At 8:30 a.m., nurses' notes record his temperature at 96.7 and at 9:15 am they record his heart rate as 120

Figure 1-1. Lewis's Story

Johnson, J.; Haskell; H; Barach, P. "The Lewis Blackman Hospital Patient Safety Act: It's Hard To Kill A Healthy 15-Year-Old." McLaughlin, C; Johnson, J.; Sollecito, W (Editors). "Implementing Continuous Quality Improvement in Health Care: A Global Casebook." Jones and Bartlett Learning, 2012.

one answers my call. Other times the receptionist answers with weary exaspera-tion, making it clear they consider our concerns a nuisance. They are busy, using this Sunday to spruce up the ward in preparation for a Joint Commission survey scheduled for the next day. The receptionist is painting decorations on the win-dows. Another nurse is updating the plates on the doors, including ours. When I go into the kitchen, I find someone has rearranged all the silverware and condiments and stacked them all in new plastic bins. For much of the afternoon, as I hunch over the bed with Lewis gripping my hand in pain, I can hear the nurses chattering and laughing in the break room.

Although we did not realize it, there was no attending or senior resi-dent surgeon present in the hospital on Sunday because of low week-end staffing. Our requests for a senior physician in the face of Lewis's increasing pain and weakness met with resistance from the nurses, who did not seem to want to call. When a doctor finally came, he was not the attending physician, but a senior surgical resident who never identified himself as such. Here is another quote from my journal:

Someone calls a doctor. I assume at the time that this is the attending physician I have requested, though I later learn he is a fourth-year general surgery resi-dent. It is some time before he arrives and when he does he is clearly coming in from outside, wearing a jacket and bringing with him a whiff of cold air. Apparently the intern is the only pediatric surgeon on duty in the hospital. And somewhere along the line my request for an attending physician has been quietly shelved. I do not know who made this decision.

The doctor is reassuring. He also thinks Lewis's pain is gas pain due to lack of motility in the intestine. Because Lewis has still not urinated, the doctor does an "in-out" urinary catheterization, thinking that this will relieve some of the pressure on the bowel. The catheterization produces a relatively small amount (c. 215 cc) of dark, concentrated urine. The doctor is a little surprised: he thinks a full bladder should have produced more urine. [Lewis had not urinated for nearly 12 hours.] I ask him about the pallor, the cold sweat, and the subnormal temperature. He says these are side effects of the medication, because Lewis is so young and "pristine." I wonder why they do not change the medication if it has such terrible side effects.

The doctor ordered a blood test (a metabolic panel) but critically, as we later learned, he omitted the complete blood count that might have shown infection or bleeding. When the test results came back, the nurse told us they showed an elevated potassium level but that it was nothing to worry about. What she did not say was that there were a number of other slightly aberrant values that, taken all together, might paint a concerning picture in a healthy young post-operative patient.

We were still worried, but we did not know what else to do. We thought we had seen the attending physician and had gone as high as we could go to address our concerns. Technicians routinely continued to record Lewis's increasingly unstable vital signs every 4 hours. There was no further assessment or intervention. But when the vital signs technician came at 8 a.m. the next morning, she was unable to get a blood pressure reading. The intern went to the operating room to ask what to do. When she came back, as we watched in increasing fear, she and the nurses spent over 2 hours trying to find a blood pressure device that would work. In all, they took Lewis's blood pressure 12 different times with seven different blood pressure cuffs and machines. At noon, shortly after another ketorolac injection, Lewis went into cardiac arrest as phlebotomists tried to draw blood for a second metabolic panel. After a slight delay, a cardiac arrest code was called. Lewis was declared dead about an hour and a half later. Again, my journal recounts the details:

We were asked to leave the room and wait in the hall. Someone comes to get us. The doctors want to talk to us. I am fearful they will tell us Lewis is brain-damaged. When we go into the room, there are five surgeons in green scrubs. One introduces himself as Dr. Adamson. He is the doctor on call. We have never seen him before. Dr. Adamson says, "We lost him." This makes no sense to me. He is speaking as though Lewis has lost a battle with a long illness. He has to repeat it several times before I understand.

The physicians told us that they did not know why Lewis died. They said their chief resident had found nothing wrong the night before. This was the first we knew that the doctor who had come the night before had not been the attending physician we had requested.

Conclusion

A month after Lewis's death, we journeyed back to the hospital to meet with the surgeon who had performed Lewis's surgery. The surgeon listened to our story with compassion; he apologized and accepted responsibility for Lewis's death. We have always admired his courage in doing this.

The hospital later settled with us without a lawsuit. A physician friend with whom we had consulted was not surprised. "It's hard to kill a healthy 15-year-old," he said. A year and a half later the attending physicians involved in Lewis's care coauthored an institutional study comparing complications of the minimally invasive surgical procedure Lewis had with the open-chest procedure that it was in the process of replacing. The study, a retrospective chart review of 116 patients having the procedure in two institutions, was terminated a few weeks before the date of Lewis's surgery and reported "no deaths" among the surgical patients (Fonkalsrud et al., 2002).

It became our mission to try to find out what had happened to take our vibrant, exuberant boy from robust health to death in just 4 days. We spent months, in some cases years, trying to follow all the threads in our son's case. When we put it all together, we realized that our son was the victim of a profoundly dysfunctional medical system. We had thought we were sophisticated consumers, but we gradually realized that we had sacrificed our firstborn child to a system whose dangers we had almost no way of knowing. The system had not malfunctioned. It was simply not designed to respond in a timely fashion to an in-hospital emergency.

Case Discussion

The tragic and needless death of Lewis Blackman can be understood in the context of errors in decision making (Acquaviva, K., Haskell, H., Johnson 2013). The autopsy identified the cause of Lewis's death as an undiagnosed perforated giant duodenal ulcer, of a type often associated with NSAIDs (Collen & Chen, 1995). As a result of the perforation, Lewis had developed peritonitis and had lost more than half his blood into his peritoneal cavity.

Lewis's parents blamed the devastating outcome on the confusion and poor communication of the teaching hospital hierarchy, and particularly on their inability to determine which caregivers were fully trained professionals and which were clinical trainees. In addition, the problem was exacerbated by lack of supervision and inability of the professionals-in-training to diagnose the real problem and intervene to save their son. No fully trained surgeon saw Lewis in the 2 days before he died.

The fatal cascade of events outlined in Lewis's case led to a legislative requirement requested by the patient advocacy group Mothers Against Medical Error (MAME). MAME worked with South Carolina hospitals to pass the Lewis Blackman Hospital Patient Safety Act. This state law requires that hospital personnel wear badges that indicate their jobs and professional status, that hospitals give patients information on the role of residents and students in their care, that patients be allowed to contact their attending physicians directly, and, that hospitals give patients and families a means of calling for immediate help in urgent medical situations. The intent of the South Carolina Department of Health and Environmental Control to enforce the law through inspection is outlined in the memorandum shown in **Exhibit 1-1**.

Subsequently, the state of South Carolina endowed the Lewis Blackman Chair of Clinical Effectiveness and Patient Safety as a testament to Lewis's remarkable young life and as a commitment to advance the health and safety of all South Carolinians. Nine simulation clinics have been established across the state for training healthcare providers in the teamwork techniques needed for dealing with emergency situations. These simulation clinics use team training exercises and sophisticated simulation technology with high-end full-body adult and infant mannequins to simulate patients with various clinical scenarios. A plaque dedicated to Lewis is featured in each of the simulation clinics.

Exhibit 1-1 Overview of Lewis Blackman Hospital Patient Safety Act

The Lewis Blackman Hospital Patient Safety Act (Article 27, Section 44-7-3410 et. seq.) was added to the SC Code of Laws, effective June 8, 2005. The act authorized the South Carolina Department of Health and Environmental Control (DHEC) to implement and enforce the provisions of the act, which requires hospitals to, among other things:

1. Identify all clinical staff, clinical trainees, medical students, interns, and resident physicians (as defined in the Act) as such with identification badges that include their names, their departments, and their job or trainee titles. All the above must be clearly visible and explicitly identified as such on their badges and must be stated in terms or abbreviations reasonably understandable;

2. Institute a procedure whereby a patient may request that a nurse call his or her attending physician (as defined in the Act) regarding the patient's personal medical care. If so requested, the nurse shall place the call and notify the physician and or his or her designee of the patient's concerns. If the patient is able to communicate with and desires to call his or her attending physician or designee (as defined in the Act), upon the patient's request, the nurse must provide the patient with the telephone number and assist the patient in placing the call;

3. Provide a mechanism available at all times, and the method for accessing it, through which a patient may access prompt assistance for the resolution of the patient's personal medical care concerns. "Mechanism" means telephone number, beeper number, or other means of allowing a patient to independently access the patient assistance system. If a patient needs assistance, a clinical staff member or clinical trainee (as defined in the Act) must assist the patient in accessing the mechanism;

4. Establish procedures for the implementation of the mechanism providing for initiation of contact with administrative or supervisory clinical staff who shall promptly assess the urgent patient care concern and cause the patient care concern to be addressed.

5. Provide to each patient prior to, or at the time of the patient's admission to the hospital for inpatient care or outpatient surgery, written information describing the general role of clinical trainees, medical students, interns, and resident physicians in patient care. This information must also:

   a. State whether medical students, interns, or resident physicians may be participating in a patient's care, may be making treatment decisions for the patient, or may be participating in or performing, in whole or in part, any surgery on the patient.

   b. Notify the patient that the attending physician is the person responsible for the patient's care while the patient is in the hospital and that the patient's attending physician may change during the patient's hospitalization.

   c. Include a description of the mechanism (see above) providing for initiation of contact with administrative or supervisory clinical staff and the method for accessing it.

Johnson, J.; Haskell, H; Barach, P. "The Lewis Blackman Hospital Patient Safety Act: It's Hard To Kill A Healthy 15-Year-Old." McLaughlin, C; Johnson, J.; Sollecito, W (Editors). "Implementing Continuous Quality Improvement in Health Care: A Global Casebook." Jones and Bartlett Learning, 2012.

Questions

1. Where did the system fail Lewis and his family?

2. Where in the process of care did incidents (errors, near misses, adverse events, and harm) occur?

3. What would be the elements of a more transparent informed consent process?

4. What aspects of this incident will the legislation cited in the case address? Which aspects does it not address, and what else should be done to prevent similar incidents?

5. What can we learn from this case in designing strategies and/ or tools to engage patients and families?

6. Which of the core competencies for health professions are most relevant for this case? Why?

References

Acquaviva, K., Haskell, H., & Johnson, J. (2013). Human cognition and the dynamics of failure to rescue: The Lewis Blackman case. *Journal of Professional Nursing, 29*(2), 95–101.

Collen, M. J., & Chen, Y. K. (1995). Giant duodenal ulcer and nonsteroidal anti-inflammatory drug use. *Am J Gastroenterol, 90*(1), 162.

Crump, H. (1992). Pectus excavatum. *American Family Physician, 46*(1), 173–179.

Fonkalsrud, E. W., Beanes, S., Hebra, A., Adamson, W., & Tagge, E. (2002). Comparison of minimally invasive and modified Ravitch pectus excavatum repair. *Journal of Pediatric Surgery, 37*(3), 413–417.

Jaroszewski, D., Notrica, D., McMahon, L., Steidley, D. E., & Deschamps, C. (2010). Current management of pectus excavatum: A review and update of therapy and treatment recommendations. *Journal of the American Board of Family Medicine, 23*(2), 230–239.

Medline. (2007). Pectus excavatum. *MedLine Plus Medical Encyclopedia.* U.S. National Library of Medicine and the National Institutes of Health.

Shamberger, R. (1996). Congenital chest wall deformities. *Current Problems in Surgery, 33*(6), 469–542.

Additional Recommended Readings

Gibson, R., & Singh, J. P. (2010). *The treatment trap.* Chicago: Ivan R. Dee.

Monk, J. (2002). How a hospital failed a boy who didn't have to die. *The State*, June 16, 2002, A1, A8–A9.

Routine Appendectomy

John's Story (Australia)

Sandra Pintabona

Editors' Note

The story of John's appendectomy is written from the perspective of his wife, Sandra Pintabona. Sandra is a clinical nurse in charge of a busy gastro-surgical ward in Perth, Western Australia, and works regularly in all patient areas. She has been nursing for over 26 years, with more than 21 years in the gastro-surgical area. At the time of John's operation, in February 2000, she had been working at a major metropolitan tertiary hospital for nearly 10 years.

An appendectomy is a common procedure consisting of the surgical removal of the vermiform appendix. Appendicitis is one of the most common surgical emergencies, and appendectomy is the treatment of choice of noncomplicated appendicitis. The procedure is normally performed as an emergency procedure. An appendectomy may be performed through a laparoscope or as an open operation. Although recovery time from the operation varies from person to person, surgical results are usually excellent with rare morbidity.

LEARNING OBJECTIVES

After completing this case study, you will be able to:

1. Outline the system failures that were evident in the care process.
2. Discuss factors related to patient and family satisfaction of care.
3. Develop a strategy for engaging the patient and family members in the care process.

John's Appendectomy

It was February 1, 2000, and I was on night duty at a major metropolitan tertiary hospital.[1] When I left for work, John was fit and well. At about 3 a.m. I received a phone call from John describing pain that fit that of appendicitis. He had a similar pain the month before that settled spontaneously. At the time, his general practitioner (GP) felt that the episode was possibly appendicitis, as his white cells were also raised, but no further workup was done. I left work immediately to assist my husband and to take him to the hospital.

We arrived at another major metropolitan tertiary hospital at about 4:20 a.m., and we were taken straight through and were seen quite quickly. The nurse took John's vital signs and asked for a sample of urine. Dr. Smith, a resident, saw John shortly afterwards at 4:30 a.m., examined him, and mentioned that there was blood in his urine sample. The doctor was concerned that he had renal colic and ordered an x-ray to rule out renal colic. John returned to the emergency room at about 5:30 a.m.; the result of the x-ray was negative for renal colic, and appendicitis was the working diagnosis. An intravenous cannula was inserted, and several doses of morphine and maxalon were given at 6:30 a.m. This made John very drowsy. He fell asleep and was difficult to arouse.

Dr. Jones, surgical registrar (team 1), arrived approximately at 7:00 a.m. and confirmed it was appendicitis. He said John required an appendectomy and that he would perform it in the late afternoon. We told Dr. Jones that we had private insurance, and Dr. Jones said that he would get Mr. Culley, the surgery consultant, to perform the surgery.[2]

As I walked out of the emergency department I saw Dr. Bone, surgical resident (team 1), enter John's cubicle. After making my phone

[1] As part of the legal settlement, John signed an agreement that he would not reveal any names of the people or institutions involved in his care. The names of the clinicians and institutions used in this case are pseudonyms.
[2] The distinction of Mr. is used by surgeons in the Australia, New Zealand, Republic of Ireland, South Africa, and some other Commonwealth countries.

calls I returned to John's cubicle, and Dr. Bone had gone. John was asleep. I later learned that the consent was signed at this point. We had understood that an open technique would be used, but subsequently the surgeon chose to use a laparoscopic approach. John had no recollection of the consent process.

The nursing staff told me that John would be transferred to the ward and taken to the operating theater in late afternoon. I asked the nursing staff to call me if any changes occurred. I was asked to sign papers, financial election, etc., and I did this on my way out at about 8:00 a.m. I told John I would return prior to the surgery later that afternoon and I went home to sleep.

I telephoned the hospital reception around 10:00 a.m. to see which ward John had been allocated and was informed that he had been taken to theater already. I returned to the hospital at 4 p.m. with our daughter. I was shocked by John's appearance. My immediate impression was that extensive surgery had been performed. His face was so pale, his lips were white—the same colour as his face. He looked severely anaemic.

John was delirious. He had a morphine patient-controlled analgesia (PCA) pump, an intravenous infusion, and an indwelling urinary catheter. I immediately looked at his abdomen, and noted a mini-laparotomy incision from belly button down to pubic bone. The wound was dry and covered with a clear plastic adhesive dressing. I saw five other small cuts on his abdomen—three on the left side, one at the navel, and one at the distal end of the laparotomy wound. The abdomen was flat with no evidence of hematoma or bruising. At this time I asked John what had happened and he didn't know, he was too drowsy.

The nurse came to take his vital signs and I asked her what was wrong with John. She said she would call the doctor to come speak with me. I was expecting Mr. Culley, but a surgical resident, Dr. Romano, surgical resident (team 2), came to speak with me instead.

I asked him what was wrong with John. He told me that it was a very difficult operation that commenced laparoscopically and was converted to an open laparotomy, and that Mr. Queen, surgeon consultant (team 2), would explain the details to me in the morning. I asked who Mr. Queen was, and Dr. Romano replied that Mr. Queen was the surgeon who did the operation. I said that I thought Mr. Culley (team 1) was to do the operation, and Dr. Romano replied that he did not know the details of why Mr. Queen had performed the operation.

At about 4:30 p.m. I noticed blood oozing from the distal end of the wound edges spreading to the left side beneath the clear plastic dressing. Several nurses came to take a look. They seemed concerned. At that time I was happy the nurses were taking appropriate action. I went home with our daughter.

Later that night my mother-in-law and brother-in-law visited John. I telephoned them when they got home. John's mother told me John's wound had broken open, was bleeding, and that it had been stitched closed. I telephoned the nurse looking after John immediately, as I was distressed that I hadn't been informed. The nurse told me that John was very agitated because his analgesia was not working. I asked if I could come sit with him if he was agitated. I was told that he was okay and that he was settled at that time.

The next morning I visited John. The nursing staff told me that his wound had dehisced as he got out of bed and that he had vomited that night. I was told that his wound was stitched closed at the bedside. John did not remember much. I asked if I could shower my husband and the nursing staff were happy for me to do this. As I showered him, I was shocked at the extensive bruising that had become apparent on his left flank and abdominal region that extended from his nipple to knee. It was very black. His scrotum and penis were at least three times their size, edematous, and black with bruising. I put John back in bed. He was exhausted, and he felt nauseated.

At 8:00 a.m. Dr. Romano, Mr. Kuhn, Mr. Queen, Dr. Thomas, and numerous medical students came to see John. Mr. Queen introduced himself and said he and Dr. Thomas had performed the operation as Mr. Culley was too busy the previous afternoon to slot John onto his surgical list. Mr. Queen said Mr. Kuhn had also assisted Dr. Thomas. The only details of the operation I was given was that it was a difficult case, there was a lot of bleeding, and the bladder was very bruised.

Mr. Queen then became aware that I knew Dr. Thomas because she recognized me. Mr. Queen asked me about my experience and where I worked. I asked for John to be transferred to a hospital closer to home, a major private hospital. Mr. Queen said he had privileges at that hospital, and he would organize the transfer himself.

I was not happy with John's condition, and I felt that something had occurred that I was not being told about; however, I reassured myself that I was told that everything would be okay and that if anything major had happened I would have been told, especially since I am part of the medical fraternity. I thought John would recover and be home in a few days. I also felt that Mr. Queen knew his case and if anything untoward occurred that he would be diligent in telling me and rectifying it promptly.

On February 2, John was transferred to a major private hospital. John progressed adequately, but slowly. Mr. Queen said he would progress slowly due to the extent of the surgery. On the morning of the third postoperative day, February 5 (a Saturday), Mr. Queen saw John again. John asked him, "Which artery did you cut to produce the extensive bruising?" Mr. Queen replied reluctantly that he had cut a mesenteric artery, but this was minor and nothing to worry about. There was no mention of a bladder trauma or perforation. A discharge date was set for the following Monday. On Sunday, John became increasingly unwell and had severe abdominal pain.

I was present on Sunday morning when Mr. Queen saw John; he stood at the foot of the bed. I noted that Mr. Queen did not examine John, and he prescribed increased doses of pethidine injection. The pain continued, and the medication did little to resolve the pain. On several occasions I expressed concerns to Mr. Queen about the intensity of the abdominal pain, suggesting that further investigation was necessary. I requested an abdominal x-ray and blood be sent. I was concerned that John was septic, because of his temperatures and wound ooze. Mr. Queen's demeanor and comments were derisive. I felt that all of my requests were treated with contempt. The only thing that I was told was that it was a normal recovery and that it was normal to be slow given the extent of the surgery, and that it would take time.

John became tachycardic, hypertensive, and febrile. His wound began to ooze further. His abdomen was distended. On Monday, February 7, John became increasingly unwell and was having rigors (shaking chills). He continued to receive pethidine injections for pain. He had explosive diarrhea and was burping fecal-smelling burps. His abdomen was making loud rumbling noises, had become increasingly distended, tympanic to percussion, and very firm to palpation. The wound continued to ooze, and dressings were applied by nursing staff. Mr. Queen spoke to John and me that morning and said, "John probably has an intestinal infection, probably *Clostridium difficile*, which is common in patients who have had surgery and are a bit run down and compromised." He ordered stool specimens to be collected. John's diarrhea stopped until the night, and at about 7 p.m. a specimen was obtained by nursing staff.

On the morning of February 8, I arrived at the hospital at about 7:30 a.m. to assist my husband in his hygiene needs. I stayed at the hospital until about 7:00 p.m. John was still obviously unwell and complaining of abdominal pain and cramping; he continued to burp copiously, foul fecal-smelling wind. He was hiccoughing continuously and very close to vomiting. His wound continued to ooze bloody-serous fluid. His abdomen was severely distended. His diarrhea had settled, but he continued to pass small amounts of wind per rectum with great difficulty and concentration. Mr. Queen arrived at about 8 a.m. and saw John from the end of the bed. He did not examine his abdomen. I expressed my concerns to Mr. Queen about the distension and pain, and my concerns were dismissed again. I tried to reassure myself that everything would be okay. I trusted the surgeon's skills and that he would be truthful with us.

Mr. Queen prescribed Imodium, and John had several doses following several small bowel movements of explosive diarrhea. As the morning progressed John became even further distended and unwell. The diarrhea stopped after the Imodium, but the pain became intolerable. The pain was cramping in nature, from one side to the other. John was not eating or taking fluids. The nurses called Mr. Queen on several occasions. At 11:00 a.m. Mr. Queen was telephoned again and an order of Buscopan 20 mg was given via a phone order. Mr. Queen never came to see John. The Buscopan did very little for the pain.

An x-ray was ordered at about 1:00 p.m., and he was taken there at 2:00 p.m. I waited for John in his room. John returned with his x-ray at about 2:30 p.m. I looked at the x-rays and report and I saw evidence of a bowel obstruction. I expected conventional treatment to be commenced (i.e., bed rest, nothing by mouth, decompression from above with either nasogastric tube or duodenal tube, and possible disimpaction). A nurse entered the room and said that she was going to ring Mr. Queen with the results. She called Mr. Queen about 3 p.m. The x-rays remained at the foot of the bed, but to my surprise Mr. Queen did not look at the x-rays.

The nurse returned and said she had spoken with Mr. Queen by phone and that John was allowed to have diet and fluids. I questioned the nurse in disbelief, and she again confirmed that John was allowed to eat and drink. The nurse seemed unconcerned. I advised John to take only fluids. He couldn't tolerate anything beyond that anyway.

I left the hospital around 4 p.m. and returned about an hour later with our daughter. John was much the same. I was told by the nursing staff that Mr. Queen had still not seen John and was not planning on coming in to see him. John was very irritable, his abdomen looked like it was going to burst, and he could not pass any wind per rectum now. At 7 p.m. I left to go home. The pain was a little better, and he seemed slightly more positive. I wasn't happy with the situation, but I was reassured by nursing staff that Mr. Queen would contact me if anything changed.

I returned home and about 5 minutes later I received a phone call from a good friend who was visiting John. He was very somber on the phone and wouldn't tell me the details. He asked me to come back to the hospital immediately. I returned to the hospital as quick as I could. I entered John's room and was shocked and distressed with what I saw. I have never seen anyone his age look so ill following an appendectomy and a bowel obstruction. I looked at his wound and a small 4 cm area had dehisced and was gaping. This was the same area that had previously dehisced. A large amount of hemo-purulent exudate was on the floor and covered his pyjamas. The wound was covered with gauze that contained a large amount of exudate. He was shaking uncontrollably, was pale, sweaty, and talking of death. He was giving his verbal and financial wishes to his friend (our accountant). I felt he was saying his last goodbyes. I couldn't help but think he wasn't going to make it out alive or at least he would need a transfer to intensive care.

Mr. Queen arrived at approximately 8:00 p.m. and spoke to me at the nurses' station. He showed me the x-ray of John's abdomen, which was taken at 2 p.m., and said the bowel was extremely distended and he required surgery immediately. I agreed to the surgery, as I felt that if it was not done as soon as possible John would be further seriously compromised.

John was seen by the anesthetist. It was necessary to do a venous cutdown to obtain a vein to administer IV fluids as John was very dehydrated, anemic, and tachycardic (180 beats per minute) and he had high blood pressure. He was given intravenous fluids and huge amounts of pethidine for the pain. Within the hour he was taken to the operating theater, and he returned 1 hour later to the ward. John had a high-grade bowel obstruction due to adhesions. On arrival he was confused; he told me he was going to get out of bed and sit on the chair. I was afraid to go home and decided to stay the night. I stayed for the next 10 nights. I was appalled that John had tension sutures on his abdomen, but happy in a way as I knew normal sutures would never hold. Mr. Queen came to see John on the ward and explained to me the procedures. He never told me that John's abdomen was full of infection and pus. Mr. Queen said that he had put tension sutures in John's abdomen so that he (Mr. Queen) would be able to sleep at night.

John remained unwell and confused overnight, He was very tachycardic, hypertensive, and he had very low oxygen saturations at 80% on room air. He had difficulty breathing and was having intense claustrophobic feelings. He had fecal fluid draining from his nasogastric tube into a bag, and it was very offensive smelling. This continued for several days. He was given routine triple broad spectrum intravenous antibiotic therapy.

John began twitching and jerking in the early morning of February 9. I expressed my concerns to a nurse that John might be reacting to the pethidine as he had had about 1500 mg within the last 24 hours. The nurse did not know what I was talking about. Several minutes later the anaesthetist walked in and I expressed my concerns to him. The pethidine was changed to morphine and midazolam and ketamine were added. The twitching took some time to settle.

On February 10, John was diagnosed with MRSA (methicillin-resistant *Staphylococcus aureas*) from intraperitoneal fluids from a sample taken during the operation. Mr. Queen said that I was the source of the infection because I worked in a "dirty hospital" (I subsequently had swabs done that were negative for MRSA, but did eventually also end up with it, probably from caring for John). He was commenced on intravenous vancomycin twice a day. I was happy with this treatment. After about five doses of vancomycin it was stopped as John's IV cannula fell out. Mr. Queen would not discuss this with me and avoided me. John still had pus exuding from his abdomen and had cellulitic areas. I requested some blood tests be done as none had been done in almost a week. A blood test was ordered by Mr. Queen on February 13. John's hemoglobin (Hb) was low, and the vancomycin levels were not even therapeutic. I mentioned the hemoglobin to Mr. Queen, but he was not concerned and said, "You don't want him to have a blood transfusion, do you?" My reply was, "He will need one if he gets any sicker." John continued to vomit and feel nauseated for days. Mr. Queen said this happened because the bowel was overdistended and edematous from the bowel obstruction.

He developed signs of another bowel obstruction; I requested an x-ray for which he obliged. An ileus was evident. Mr. Queen decided to give John Gastrografin orally on February 14 to try to resolve this, but he continued to vomit. John required constant antiemetics and intravenous hydration until February 17, when he was finally able to hold down fluids in small amounts.

On February 15, Mr. Queen informed John that he was travelling interstate, and that another surgeon would take over his care. By this point, John and I had lost all confidence in Mr. Queen and his associates. I disengaged Mr. Queen as the treating surgeon via a phone call directly and engaged the care of another surgeon whom I had worked with for many years. Mr. Queen apologized to us for what had happened.

The next morning our new surgeon came to see John. He palpated, percussed, and auscultated John's abdomen. This was the first time I had seen this done since John's time in the emergency department. Our new surgeon contacted microbiology and commenced appropriate antibiotics, a further swab was taken, and he saw John twice a day. The intravenous fluids were continued, and routine daily blood tests were taken. John progressed slowly, but we were very happy with the treatment, and we had confidence in our new surgeon. John was discharged from hospital on February 21 to home nursing, approximately 3 weeks after his appendectomy. He needed ongoing wound care for his tension sutures that remained in for 3 weeks.

John finally returned to work after several months, but he continued to have infectious draining from the distal end of his wound. He finally healed but abscesses broke out a year later that proved to be due to a MRSA infection. John required a further laparotomy due to a large incisional hernia and a massive ventral defect. This was repaired in December 2001 with mesh as there was not enough muscle to close the defect and a large bulging area was still evident.

Conclusion

During the past 10 years, John has continued to suffer from intermittent bowel obstruction caused by the adhesions. He has also suffered from urinary bladder problems. Subsequent to legal action we found out that his bladder had been perforated during the appendectomy and an artery had been severed during the procedure. John had been given 6 to 8 liters of intravenous fluid preoperatively, for which the hospital did not monitor on a preoperative check. So John went into the theater with a full bladder. It was not hospital policy to monitor or document the amount of intravenous fluid input and urine output within the emergency department. When the surgeon inserted his instruments into the abdomen, the bladder was very distended. It was perforated and injured, and a subsequent hemorrhage occurred.

Case Discussion

This is an unfortunate and complex story in which a patient had serious complications and long-lasting morbidity due to neglect and misunderstanding of clinical signs and symptoms that pointed to his underlying pathology. The trust of the patient and family were seriously eroded when a series of unplanned and unexpected injuries to the patient's bladder and mesenteric artery during the surgical procedure were not disclosed to the patient or family in a timely manner. The lack of timely and unambiguous communication with the wife coupled with a rude, insulting, and derisive demeanor further resulted in patient harm, family unhappiness, and loss of trust. A series of contributory factors influenced and created the conditions that led to a series of adverse processes and outcomes of care.

The system failed the patient and family in spite of many opportunities to intervene and attend to the patient. The patient's wife was a seasoned nurse and therefore had valuable insights and perspective; however, her insights were neglected or even derided. The family was very unhappy with the care, which led to the ultimate dismissal of the care provider. We know that overall patient and family satisfaction is tied to the following factors (Boulding et al., 2011):

- Communication with nurses
- Pain management
- Timeliness of assistance
- Explanation of medications administered
- Communication with doctors

Although there are unresolved methodological issues related to the measurement and interpretation of patient experiences—regarding survey content, risk adjustment, and the mode and timing of survey administration—theory and the available evidence suggest that such measures are robust, distinctive indicators of healthcare quality (Manary et al., 2013). The debate could center not on whether patients can provide meaningful quality measures, but on how to improve patient experiences. This could be done by focusing on activities such as care coordination and patient engagement found to be associated with both satisfaction and outcomes.

Questions

1. How would you rate the care from the patient and provider perspectives?

2. What were the system failures in John's care?

3. What are the human factors and social-technical factors that contributed to the patient's adverse course?

4. What could the patient or family have done during this case to help prevent this outcome?

5. What can we learn from this case in designing strategies and/ or tools to empower patients and families?

6. Do patients' reports of their healthcare experiences reflect the quality of care?

7. Which of the core competencies for health professions are most relevant for this case? Why?

References

Boulding, W., Glickman, S. W., Manary, M. P., Schulman, K. A., & Staelin, R. (2011). Relationship between patient satisfaction with inpatient care and hospital readmission within 30 days. *American Journal of Managed Care*, *17*(1), 41–48.

Manary, M. P., Boulding, W., Staelin, R., & Glickman, S. W. (2013). The patient experience and health outcomes. *New England Journal of Medicine*, *368*(3), 201–203.

The Origins of the Mid Staffordshire Inquiry into the National Health Service

The Story of Bella Bailey

Julie Bailey (United Kingdom)

Editors' Note

Julie Bailey is from Stafford, in the middle of England, between Birmingham and Manchester. She grew up in Stafford, and her adult children and granddaughter live nearby. Julie's mother, Bella Bailey, was 86 years old when she was admitted to the hospital in 2007 with a hiatal hernia. Bella's experience and untimely death, and Julie's observation of care in the hospital, ultimately led to the Mid Staffordshire Inquiry, which brought about great changes in the way care is provided under the British National Health Service (Mid Staffordshire NHS Foundation Trust, 2013).

LEARNING OBJECTIVES

After completing this case study, you will be able to:

1. Describe the system failures that led to Bella Bailey's death and subsequently to the Mid Staffordshire Inquiry.
2. Create a strategy for hospital public accountability.
3. Develop an action plan to improve workplace culture.

My Mother and My Best Friend

My mother was 86 years old and was in poor health. She lived with me for the last 2 years of her life, and when people say your mum is your best friend . . . my mother really *was* my best friend. She was born in London and was proper Cockney. She served during the war in the WAAF, the Women's Auxiliary Air Force.

Despite all her illnesses she was a strong character, and she was the type of person who was the life and soul of the party. She was admitted to the hospital with a hiatal hernia. She had complained about the problem for about 6 months, and it had restricted her swallowing to the point where she was on a soft diet. She had a lot of soup and porridge, but she was a bit of a rebel as well. She had eaten tomatoes that had affected her hiatal hernia. That was really why she went into the hospital: the tomatoes had inflamed the hernia, causing her great pain and discomfort.

Staffordshire General Hospital

Mum was admitted to Staffordshire General Hospital straight onto the ward because the doctor had admitted her from home. (The process map in **Figure 3-1** provides an overview of Bella's inpatient journey.) At that time, I quickly realized that she was developing a chest infection. She was prone to these infections. I knew the signs, and we had a certain routine where she would be given antibiotics and steroids, and that usually relieved the infection. But trying to get the doctors to listen to me was really difficult. They kept strapping her up to the heart monitor because she had pain in her chest and their main concern was heart attack.

Eventually, on the third day, I collected her sputum overnight and showed the doctor, and as soon as I did that they could see there was a problem. She had the first dose of antibiotics on her fourth day of the admission. Later that day, a nurse appeared and said that

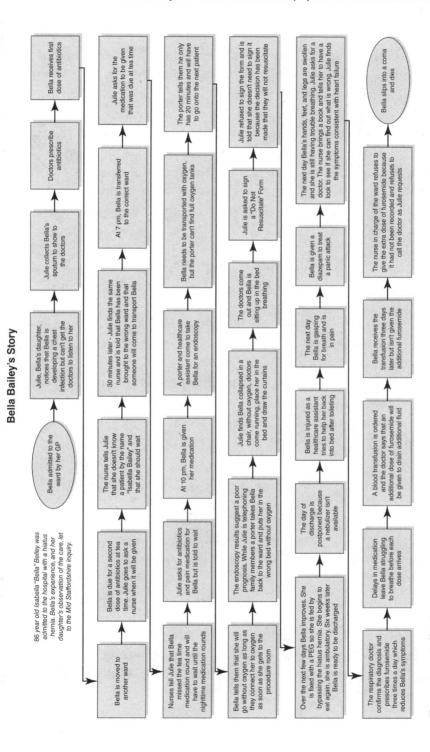

Figure 3-1. Bella's Story

31

they were moving my mother to a different ward. So we bundled everything up and off we went. We got to the new ward and we walked into the room; it was a four-bed room and there was just one little lady sitting there.

I said hello to the lady but she did not reply, and I quickly realized that the lady was confused. She just sat there with a summer dress on and no shawl, not looking up or responding to me at all. After 3 hours of us sitting in the room, me in a chair and my mother in the bed, a healthcare assistant came in to place a food tray down for the elderly lady.

As she walked out of the room I said, "Excuse me, is anybody coming to see to my mother? We have been here nearly 3 hours."

She said, "I am on dinner service. I have nothing to do with people coming and going; I only serve dinners." And off she trotted.

After about 20 minutes she came back into the room and picked up the tray. I said to the assistant that the lady had not touched her food. Her response was, "She never does," and she went to leave the room.

So I asked, "Will a nurse be coming to see to my mother?"

I was aware that Mother had just had one dose of antibiotics and she was due for a second dose at teatime. I was concerned because this infection had been now for at least 4 days, and I was anxious for this medication to be given.

I went out into the corridor. Eventually a nurse came by, so I ran out to her and asked her about my mother's medication. The nurse asked who my mother was and I said her name and she said she did not know of anybody by the name of Isabella Bailey. She told me to wait.

About a half an hour later I went back out again and when I found the nurse she said that we had been brought to the wrong ward. My answer was, "Will we be going to the right ward?" and her response was, "Yes we will get somebody to take you."

So we waited and waited until about 7 o'clock and two nurses came in and wheeled my mother over to Ward 11. As I was walking down the ward there were people standing all along the corridor, relatives waiting outside each door, and the noise was just horrendous. There were patients shouting out to the nurses, and it just seemed like chaos that we were going into.

Ward 11

The nurses wheeled Mum into her room and transferred her into her bed, and as the nurses were about to leave I asked if Mum could have her teatime medication that she was due.

The nurse said, "No. You are late. We were ready for you at teatime. You will have to wait until the nighttime medication round."

I replied that our being late had nothing to do with us, we had been taken to the wrong ward. She said, "It is not my problem," and just walked off.

The woman in the next bed to my mother was screaming. For that first night all she did was scream out in pain and nobody would come to her. She kept pressing the buzzer and eventually a woman walked down the ward with a suit on—she was not a nurse—and she burst into the room and said to the woman, "Look, what you need to understand is that there is no need for you to worry. There is nothing wrong with you. Your problem is, you are used to being in charge, but now you are not in charge. We are in charge of this ward, not you. There is nothing wrong with you; you have been seen by three different doctors." And then out she walked.

This poor woman was just hysterical in the bed and so I went over to her and asked her if I could do anything. She explained to me that she had been a nurse in Manchester and she believed she had a clot in her leg, but she could not get them to accept what was going on. She had been seen by three doctors, but she said they were all junior doctors and they did not understand what was going on.

I did not want to go back to the nurses' station as I did not know what they would say, but I just had to. The woman was holding onto the bed bars, she was in so much pain. My mum was in pain as well with her chest. I asked if there was any way we could get her medication. The nurse said that the woman had been seen by the doctor and it was really not anything to do with me.

I said, "But Mum needs some pain relief and her antibiotics, too." The nurse said, "The drug round will be around at 10 o'clock." So I went back to my mum and waited and waited. When 10 o'clock came, she finally got her medication.

The next day I went back and the woman in the bed had been seen by a doctor from another hospital. It turns out that she had called her own doctor. That doctor, a senior doctor from another hospital, had spoken to a junior doctor on the ward and she had been given the correct medication. The senior doctor told her that if she hadn't been given the medication when she was, she might have lost her leg. So for the next couple of days I was really concerned about the care my mother was receiving, but at the same time, I did not feel I could stay any longer than the visiting times.

Without Oxygen

On the fifth day I was sitting with Mum and a porter came along with a healthcare assistant and said they were taking her down to have an endoscopy. Mum needed oxygen for this procedure, and they kept bringing oxygen supplies to her, but they were all empty; they could not get one that had any oxygen in it. While this was all happening, the porter told us that he only had 20 minutes between picking up patients and he had to go to another patient.

Mum said, "Don't worry; I do not want to get you in trouble. I will go without oxygen, as long as you connect me as soon as I get down there," which they promptly did.

Mum had the endoscopy and while she was in the recovery position the doctor called me over and said, "It is a poor prognosis. The hernia is quite enlarged and it is restricting your mother's swallowing."

I was upset with this prognosis and I did not want Mum to see me crying. So I asked the healthcare assistant to take her back up and to tell her that I would be back in 15 minutes. I went outside and phoned my niece. I told her what had happened and asked her to come and see Mum and just keep her company, and that I would come up once I felt a little bit stronger. So my niece came and went up to visit my mother.

After the endoscopy there was no healthcare assistant available to take Mum back to her room. Eventually a porter had to bring her back. My niece did not know where Mum's bed was or where she should have been. So the porter just left her without any oxygen supply. My niece asked if they could reconnect the oxygen and the porter said the nurse would be with them shortly. My niece waited and eventually my mother collapsed onto the chair. My niece had been out in the hall asking for help and they kept saying they would be with her in a minute.

My niece immediately rang me and said, "Julie, come quick; I think we are going to lose Mother." I came running up the stairs and saw her collapsed in the chair. I ran out into the hall and some doctors came running and asked if she was breathing. They placed her into a bed and drew the curtains. Within a few minutes the doctors came out and Mother was sitting up in the bed breathing.

The doctor said that he needed to speak to me. He took me into a room and he said, "I need you to sign this form."

I said, "What is it?"

He said, "It is a Do Not Resuscitate form."

I said, "What do you mean? I have just nearly lost my mum and you have nearly left her to die in the chair."

He said that was nothing to do with them, that was the nursing staff. I said, "I am sorry. I am not signing this form."

He said, "Look, your mum is going to have a painful death. She is going to die over the weekend and the best thing you can do is go home and leave her here with us."

I could not believe what he was telling me. I ran out of the room and said to my niece, "Come and listen to this!" and the doctor just repeated it in exactly the same words to us both.

I ran out into the ward; I was so upset. Another doctor came and pulled me into a room and I said, "I cannot believe what I have just heard."

He said, "We do not need you to sign the Do Not Resuscitate. We are making the decision. We are not going to resuscitate her."

I said, "This is not about that. I want to know that my mum is going to get pain relief. I have had a struggle the last 4 days. My mum is going to die a painful death and I just want something to relieve her of that pain."

I decided from that point on I was not going to leave my mum's side.

Confused Patients

Patients were wandering around the ward. Several of the patients were confused, but the staff did not seem to have the skills to manage that. They would shout at the patients and the patients would get angry. There were no pillows, no blankets; the patients were cold. There was no help to feed them or help them to the toilet. I even saw patients drinking from vases at night because there were no water drinks left out. It really was a frightening situation.

I sat on the chair all night next to Mum's bed. I would wedge down the curtains with chairs to try and stop people from coming in, because very often you would wake up and there would be some man over you. I was petrified, and I was a well person.

Despite all this, Mum managed to overcome all this. They fitted a PEG feeding tube so it could bypass the hiatal hernia and she could be fed through the PEG. Also, she began to eat again so the hiatal hernia must have reduced. She was up and walking about. She was going to the toilet. She was eating again and she was ready to go home.

There was one point where a confused patient came into our room and he was violent to one of the patients. Another patient decided that she could bear it no more, and that she was going to sign herself out. As this woman started to pack she just collapsed onto the floor. As I ran over to help her, the confused patient grabbed my mother and was pulling her out of her bed, saying it was his bed. Mum was screaming to me to drop the other patient and help her. I just thought at that moment that I had had enough of all of this. So I wrote a letter to the chief executive. The letter said, "Please help us with taking care of my mother. This is dangerous. Something serious is going to happen in this hospital." I put the letter through the chief executive's door in his office hoping that he would get it, but nothing ever came of it. I did not receive a response.

However, after I made the complaint, the staff were just terrible toward us. They took the blankets that I used at night. People who had been pleasant now ignored us. I went to the toilet one night at 3:00 a.m. and they came and took all the chairs out of the room so I had to stand or sit on the bottom of my mother's bed all night and day. So we decided just to keep our heads down and rotate duties amongst my daughter and niece. I told them let's do what best we can and not upset the staff. We just kept to ourselves and we did not say anything to anyone.

Heart Failure

After 6 weeks, Mum was due to be discharged on a Friday. I had gone home and got her clothes and as I got her up walking down to the toilet the doctor called me in and said, "There has been a hold-up. We cannot send your mother home without a nebulizer."

I had never heard before that my Mum needed a nebulizer or I would have gotten one for her. He said, "We will get her a nebulizer and she will be discharged on Monday."

On the Saturday before Mum was to be discharged home my niece took over. My mother at that time needed somebody on either side of her to help her onto the bed. Normally, the healthcare assistant would help me get her onto the bed, but my niece had just found out she was pregnant and I told her not to do it. So during that night, Saturday night, my niece was asleep on the chair. One member of the staff had helped my mother onto the toilet and she tried to put my mother back into bed alone. She dropped my mother and Mum's back hit the iron bars of the bed.

My mother shouted out as she hit the bars and my niece woke up. Mum was dazed on the bed lying across the bed sort of half on the floor. Within a few minutes Mum came around again and she was shouting, "Help! Help!" When my niece asked for the doctor the nursing staff told her that there was no doctor available.

The next day when I came back my mum could not breathe. I had no clue what had happened. A nurse came and gave my mother diazepam to calm her. They said she was having a panic attack, which at the time did seem like a panic attack. She was gasping, and it was not normal for my mum to be gasping like this. The diazepam had an awful effect on her. She was confused, and she did not recognize me; it seemed to make things worse. Monday night once again Mum could not breathe so they gave her another diazepam.

The next morning I noticed Mum was all swollen, both her hands and legs. The nurse said it was because she had been lying in the bed for the past 6 weeks. It had now been 3 days since my Mum had fallen. Although a call had been made, she hadn't been seen by a doctor. One of the kinder nurses came and told me she was going home but there still wasn't a doctor available. The nurse went out of the room and returned with a big medical book, and told me to have a look through to see if I could find out what was wrong with my mother. Looking through the book, I could see straight away what was wrong. The symptoms were there in the book—it was heart failure.

Eventually that day Mum was seen by a respiratory doctor. He examined her and said that she had heart failure. He prescribed furosemide, a diuretic, and within 20 minutes she could breathe better again. All those days she had suffered and finally she was given the drug and she could breathe freely.

They said they were trying to get the medication dose right. They prescribed her medication three times a day, but by the time it was due she would start to pant again and could not breathe. There was no routine in place because they were so short-staffed, and very often the drugs were given much later than they were due. All I could do was just try and talk my mum through this horrible time and get her to breathe while we waited for her medication, but as soon as she had her drugs it was eased.

Extra Furosemide

Then they said they had taken blood tests and Mum would need a blood transfusion. The doctor came and said they would try to eliminate the risks, that they would give the transfusion to her very slowly over a period of time and would give her an extra dose of furosemide to drain away the additional fluid that accrues after the blood transfusion.

The next day, when she was due for the blood transfusion, no blood came. The following day they said the blood had arrived, but there was not enough staff to go downstairs to get it. On the third day I asked again if Mum was going to have the blood transfusion and I was once again told that there was not enough staff available to get the blood. At 4 o'clock I went home for a shower, and while I was gone my daughter rang and said that they had started the blood transfusion. So I raced back to the hospital. I got back in about 15 minutes and the blood had already gone through. I thought that was strange, as I had been told that it would go through very slowly to eliminate the risk of too much fluid on her damaged heart.

After the blood transfusion Mum still had not received the extra furosemide and she was starting to gasp once again for air and could not breathe. By this time her actual dose of the furosemide was due as well. While Mother gasped and gasped for air we just sat there unable to do anything to help her.

Three hours later, the night nurse came along, and she told us that Mother was not going to get an extra furosemide because there was no doctor's order recorded for an extra dose. The nurse was adamant that my mother was not having the extra furosemide. I realized there must have been a mistake, because I had been there when the doctor had explained the process and ordered the extra furosemide. I asked for a doctor so that he could once again prescribe this to her. The nurse placed her hands on her hips and told me that she was in charge of this ward and she would say if a doctor is called.

I have never felt this angry and bitter towards somebody before. My mum was desperate and there was nothing I could do. I thought it best if I went home, out of the way of this nurse. I rang my daughter and asked if she would stay the night instead. My daughter asked again for the extra furosemide and the nurse agreed to call a doctor. But at 5 o'clock in the morning my daughter called to tell me to hurry to the hospital, that Mum was very ill and still hadn't been seen by the doctor. When I returned she was still breathing, but unconscious. A different nurse was giving her furosemide through her feeding tube, but by now it was too late. While they were giving her the extra furosemide, she died.

I started to leave the ward. One kind doctor came and told me he was sorry for what had happened. I told him it had nothing to do with him, he did the best he could, but others hadn't and instead they had caused her death. They had left her begging for her life when they should have been looking after her. I walked out of the ward with my daughter and went straight to the church. I just sat in the church. I did not know what to do or what I could do anymore. I was totally confused. I thought about all the patients I had left behind.

Cure the NHS

I returned home and knew that I would have to do something and that I could not allow the situation to continue. The next day I contacted the director of nursing. She would not accept what I was telling her. She told me, "There is nothing wrong at this hospital. The staff are well trained. I walk the wards at night and I have never seen anything like that before." She was totally in denial.

I wrote a letter to the local newspaper and asked if there were other people in the community who had experienced poor care at the hospital, because I thought that if I had seen this it must have happened to other people as well. I received about 50 letters, all saying the same thing. All had seen neglect, lack of adequate fluid, lack of food, and indifference. Pain relief was a huge problem. I wrote a complaint letter to the hospital leadership and the reply was to say we are really sorry you feel that your mother's care was not what you expected and we will make sure that it never happens again. There was no indication of how they were going to make sure it never happened again. I filed a complaint using the second stage of the National Health Service (NHS) complaints procedure. They said that because I had suffered no hardship they would not be upholding my mother's case. They said that they contacted the hospital and there was an action plan in place to ensure that what happened to my mum did not happen again to other patients.

By this time I actually had two boxes full high of action plans that had come from other families' complaints to the hospital, so I knew the complaints procedure was pretty meaningless. One family was assured that an action plan would be implemented on Ward 11 to stop the neglect their mother had suffered some months earlier. The plan was allegedly implemented 2 weeks before my mother's admission to the same ward. Three years after my mum's death there was another patient with an almost identical case recorded in the local paper. This patient had also had a bad outcome involving the need for furosemide after a blood transfusion, so I know no lessons had been learned.

I formed a group called Cure the NHS and held meetings to discuss our concerns and to plan a way forward to alter the neglect within the hospital. When I first set up the group, the first year that the Health Care Commission investigated, it was just an awful period. Stafford is a small town, and the hospital is one of the major employers within the town. I lost all my business at the café that I owned and ran. I received anonymous phone calls and death threats. I would get to work and there would be bad things written on my café's windows and my car would be scraped and my tires slashed. The worst of it all was the menacing calls because, to be honest, I did not know what they would do. The calls stopped after the 2009 Health Care Commission report came out and confirmed that my complaints were widespread and accurate. I have never been able to build up the business again.

Conclusion

I think Cure the NHS has been effective in challenging the NHS and enabling and empowering people to support their loved ones. We put forward in our recommendations that safe staffing levels are required and that an adequate skill mix is needed within the NHS. The Mid Staffordshire Foundation Trust had a 60/40 split; that is, 60% of the healthcare staff were assistants and 40% were qualified nursing staff. The director of nursing for the NHS, when she gave evidence to the public inquiry, said she had never heard of a skill mix in which healthcare assistants were the majority.

We have tried as a group to push the NHS to be transparent with the public, so that everything that goes on in a hospital is shared with the public. I found over the years working with the public inquiry that the amount of data that is collected is phenomenal. There are certain things—complaints, serious untoward incidents, peer review reports, mortality statistics, staff surveys, patient surveys, infection rates, staff sickness rates, staffing levels, and a few other things—if you take all that data together it gives you an idea of what is going on in that hospital at a given time. If all that data had been available to the public there is no way I would have put my mother into the hospital she was in. If I had had the choice I would have placed my mother in a different hospital, one that was showing better performance indicators.

Case Discussion

In 2009, a highly critical report by the Health Care Commission (HCC) in the United Kingdom revealed a catalog of substandard care failings at the two hospitals in Mid Staffordshire and said that the appalling standards put patients at risk. According to the HCC, between 400 and 1200 more people died than would have been expected from 2005 to 2008. In February 2010, an independent inquiry led by Robert Francis, Queen's Counsel, found the hospitals had "routinely neglected patients." The public inquiry, which was commissioned in 2010, had a much wider remit. The £11 million inquiry examined what went wrong at the trust between January 2005 and March 2009. The inquiry heard from more than 150 witnesses between November 2010 and December 2011. The report was released in 2013 (Mid Staffordshire NHS Foundation Trust, 2013).

The findings of the Francis inquiry into the failings of care at Mid Staffordshire echo loudly the findings of the Bristol inquiry 10 years earlier (Dyer, 2001). These inquiries found that during the periods under investigation many staff, patients, and management had raised concerns about the standard of care provided to patients. The tragedy was that they were ignored and the concerns were covered up. Senior managers seemed more concerned about protecting their reputation than about the lives of patients in the systems under their oversight. Finally, and perhaps of most concern, these public reports found a widespread culture of denial, a lack of attentiveness to patient concerns, and normalized deviance.

The Francis inquiry became the single most important healthcare reform document for the NHS. Healthcare systems around the world looked to the NHS for guidance and monitored their actions in addressing the report's recommendations. The report called on patients to understand the impact of their disease and treatment. The report argued that clinicians and patients need to work in partnership. If we are to improve health care, we need to challenge deeply ingrained practices and behaviors.

Questions

1. What system failures were apparent in Bella Bailey's case?

2. What could family members have done to help their loved one get the right care at this hospital?

3. What needs to change to ensure that a hospital like this one delivers safe and high-quality care?

4. What can you say about the culture at this hospital?

5. Staffing levels and skill mixes in hospitals were among the first issues that Julie Bailey's advocacy organization wanted to address. Staffing ratios are highly controversial—how important are they to ensuring safe patient care? Why do you think that patients would see them as so important?

6. Julie Bailey's description of her mother's trip to the endoscopy unit paints a picture of missing supplies and confused communication. Handovers and transport of patients can be major sources of patient harm—how can this be addressed?

7. What can we learn from this case in designing strategies and/or tools to empower patients and families?

8. Of the core competencies for health professions, which do you think are most relevant for this case? Why?

References

Dyer, C. (2001). Bristol inquiry condemns hospital's "club culture." *BMJ*, *323*(7306), 181.

Mid Staffordshire NHS Foundation Trust. (2013). *Report of the Mid Staffordshire NHS Foundation Trust public inquiry*. United Kingdom: The Stationery Office Limited.

Consent and Disclosure in Pediatric Heart Surgery

The Story of James Mannix (United States)

Mary Ellen Mannix

Editors' Note

Mary Ellen Mannix and her husband Michael learned from a prenatal echocardiogram that their fourth child, James, had a high chance of being born with a heart defect—a coarctation of the aorta. The baby otherwise appeared to be healthy. The pediatric cardiologist told the couple that the diagnosis could not be confirmed until delivery and that the treatment at that time would probably be relatively straightforward—either drug therapy, balloon dilatation, or an operation to repair the aorta. "We are not talking open heart surgery here," said the doctor. When James was born, it was confirmed that he had a discrete aortic coarctation, a relatively mild form of the defect. What follows is Mary Ellen's story of what happened after James's diagnosis.

Coarctation of the aorta is one of the more common congenital defects, accounting for 5–10% of all congenital heart disease and occurring in 1 in every 1000 births. It is characterized by a narrowing of the aorta in the area of the ductus arteriosus, a fetal blood vessel conduit between the pulmonary artery and the aortic arch that normally closes shortly after birth. Prenatal detection of aortic coarctation, although highly desirable, carries a high possibility of error. Mild cases may not be detectable prenatally, and some people may not show symptoms until middle age. In more severe cases, an infant may appear healthy until several days after birth, when the closing of the ductus arteriosus can lead to diminished blood flow, heart failure, and shock (Matsui & Gardiner, 2009; Gargiulo et al., 2008).

The usual treatment for an infant diagnosed with aortic coarctation is surgery. Newborns with an unclear diagnosis may be observed in the hospital for several days, whereas a baby with a confirmed diagnosis is likely to be stabilized on medication (prostaglandin) until surgery can be performed. The repair of a discrete coarctation, like the one James had, is usually accomplished through an incision in the left side of the chest called a posterolateral thoracotomy and does not entail cardiopulmonary bypass. In more complex presentations, the child may be placed on cardiopulmonary bypass to repair the coarctation and accompanying heart defects in a single operation through a sternal incision. Mortality in surgical repair of aortic coarctation is generally reported to be low (less than 1%) (Rosenthal, 2005).

LEARNING OBJECTIVES

After completing this case study, you will be able to:

1. Examine the risk management issues around prenatal diagnosis of major cardiac defects.

2. Recognize how communication between parents and providers can be effective or ineffective in ensuring full understanding of the case ramifications.

3. Outline the risks for surgical procedures in infants.

4. Discuss how effective and authentic consent and communication between providers and patients and their families can contribute to reliable healthcare outcomes.

A Big Baby

James was delivered at 39 weeks in a planned delivery. He was the largest of my babies, weighing 8 pounds, 4 ounces and measuring 21.5 inches. He had a raspy cry, a full head of hair, and very light eyebrows. The obstetric team was surprised that he was so big because babies with heart defects tend to be small. They immediately took him to the warming table to assess him and they told me he looked great. He had high APGAR[1] scores of 9 and 10, but because he had the prenatal diagnosis of coarctation of the aorta they wanted

---

[1] The APGAR score is determined by evaluating the newborn baby on five criteria on a scale from 0 to 2, then summing up the five values obtained. The resulting APGAR score ranges from 0 to 10. The five criteria are **A**ppearance, **P**ulse, **G**rimace, **A**ctivity, and **R**espiration.

to perform an echocardiogram in the neonatal intensive care unit (NICU). We were told that as soon as they were finished we would see our baby.

Four hours went by. Finally my husband found a wheelchair, put me in it, and we made our way over to the NICU. As we approached the NICU we saw an isolette heading out. It was our son. They were about to transfer him to the pediatric heart center without telling us. At that point, we had some discussion with the pediatric cardiologist who confirmed that there was a discrete, or simple, coarctation of the aorta. James was breathing well on room air and he was not in urgent need of anything. The physician told us, "If he were my child, I would want him down there," referring to the pediatric heart center, so off he went. My understanding was that this was only for monitoring.

Is There Anything We Should Know?

I joined James at the heart center a day later. He was on room air. He was eating from a bottle. He was not in distress. That night my husband signed a consent form for repair of the aorta coarctation. Our understanding was that this meant either a pharmaceutical intervention like digoxin or possibly some kind of catheterization to balloon open the narrowing of the aorta, which was terrifying enough in itself. The surgeon was a world-famous pediatric heart surgeon. I remember asking him specifically, "Is there anything besides general anesthesia that you will be doing that we should know about?" He replied, "No, nothing at all."

We handed James off and waited. Later that day when we finally saw him he was intubated. He had a scar running down the middle of his chest. He had tubes coming out of the side of him. No one had told me or prepared me that this was a condition that I could possibly see my son in at 2 days of age. I felt stupid. I did not question it, but did ask, "What now?" The nurse said, "Well, the next time you come back to see him you will probably be able to breast-feed him, because we are going to take the breathing tube out."

At that time we had to leave because we were not allowed to be in the pediatric cardiac intensive care unit (PCICU) until visiting hours. They were very prescriptive about when we could be with our son. It was late in the day, but visiting hours did not begin until the end of rounds at 8:00 p.m. At 7:40 I remember looking at the clock and knowing that I needed to be with him right then and could not wait anymore. My husband called the PCICU to say that we would like to come down and see our son, at which time they told us that it was not a good time, and that they would call to tell us when we could come down.

A Sudden and Serious Event

A few minutes later there was a knock on the door. It was a physician and a nurse, neither of whom I had ever seen before. They told us there had been a very sudden and serious event, and they repeated those words again. I tried to ask them several times in different ways, "What does that mean? What happened?" They would only say that it was very sudden and very serious, and they ended with, "We will let you know when you can come see him." This was around 8 o'clock in the evening. It was after midnight when they called the room and said that we could come see him.

When I saw my son, he had a breathing tube taped very tightly on his mouth. His chest was open. There were tubes coming directly out of the center of my son's chest. There was a square elastic transparent bandage over his heart, and that was all there was between me and his heart. He was positioned more like a frog than the "powerhouse" picture I had taken of him as a newborn. He had a strange grayish-green color. There was blood all over the isolette.

Somebody asked if we would like a priest. I said no. I was not ready to go to where I think they wanted me to go. My husband wanted to know what had happened and again all they would say was that it was a sudden event and a very serious event.

They had him connected to life support on an ECMO machine.[2] James spent Friday, Saturday, and Sunday on the ECMO machine. On Monday morning when I saw that he was not attached to anything I nearly passed out, because I thought he was dead. They told me not to worry, that he was off ECMO and was just on the ventilator.

He was ventilated for the rest of that week, Monday through Friday, and he died on Saturday as a consequence of a ventilator-associated pneumothorax, a hole in the lung that is caused by being on the ventilator.

Insult to the Brain Stem

The day before the pneumothorax showed up the nurses started asking me questions. "Do any of your children have epilepsy? Do you have any seizure disorders?" They said they had noticed my son did this little shaking thing. I had noticed it, too. They ordered a neurologist consult. My husband left to take care of our other children, and I was alone to receive the consult information from the neurologist.

The neurologist said, "Your son has suffered serious insult to his brain stem and his cortex. He was clearly born brain healthy and something happened either during or after surgery."

I could not understand, it and the neurologist repeated himself a few times. He was sitting with me in the room and writing things down I had told him.

I said, "I work with special kids. If this means I have to work a little extra with him, I can. He will be able to crawl, right?"

---

[2] Extracorporeal membrane oxygenation (ECMO) provides both cardiac and respiratory support to patients whose heart and lungs are so severely distressed or damaged that they can no longer serve their function.

The neurologist said, "Mrs. Mannix, your son suffered serious insult to his brain stem and his cortex."

He wrote it down so I could look it up. Then he ordered a reduction in the medications my son was on, which were mainly paralytics. After they were reduced James started to open his eyes and was more reactive. They finally asked for some breast milk for him, which I had been expressing the whole time. I was pretty much filling up the unit's freezer with my breast milk, to the point that they had to ask me to please find somewhere else to store it. But James did get to have some breast milk in those few hours.

When the crisis came the next day, I had left James to go rest. I was very specific and told them that if anything happened they were to come get me. When they knocked on the door and woke me up, they said the surgeon had taken my son for emergency surgery to address the pneumothorax.

At that point, probably after the conversation with the neurologist, I had crossed a bridge. I asked why they had taken him for surgery and said I did not want them to do anything more to him. I told them that he had suffered enough, he had three siblings who wanted to meet him and hold him, and as a mom I was lucky enough to be there when he was born and I wanted to help make the transition into whatever his next life was going to be. I wanted less pain for him than what clearly this life had been.

The Size of a 9-Month-Old

This conversation took place around 7 o'clock in the morning and yet I found out later from the records that he actually did not go into surgery until 11 o'clock that morning.

When they called us to come see him after surgery, the PCICU doors opened wide and there in front of me were all the blue scrubs circling the isolette that contained my son. As I walked over to him,

I saw that he was swollen to the size of a nine month old. He was black, blue, and purple. His hand was in a fist and was completely black. They had performed a thoracotomy to repair the pneumothorax and while they were in there they had revised the coarctation repair they had done the previous week. To do this they had put him back on ECMO. Once again, he had tubes coming out of his chest.

I knew as soon as I saw my son in that state that he was gone. He was dead. And yet a nurse brings over a little tub of baby bath for me to give him a bath, because he still had blood on his chest and the side of his arm. I never dared to lift the blanket on the side where the open surgical wound was, and where the wound was still draining.

My husband asked where the surgeon was. The social worker replied that he had left his assistant there to answer our questions. At this point, that was not enough for us. Fortunately for us, or unfortunately for the surgeon, we ran into him in the hallway. He was already out of his hospital scrubs and in street clothes.

My husband asked him what had happened and who was overseeing the care over the weekend to coordinate all these different pieces to manage our son's condition. The surgeon told us that he did not work on the weekend and would not be available to talk with us. My husband asked again who would be there overseeing our son's care. The surgeon did not know. His response was, "What difference will knowing that make now?" With that, the surgeon walked away.

"You Trusted Us"

We spent 24 hours watching our son in that shape and after a conversation with the same pediatric cardiologist who had said "we were not talking open heart surgery here," my husband asked him, "You know, it was just a couple of months ago that you were telling us that this was nothing for us to worry about, that this was not a big concern. What happened?" The cardiologist's reply was, "You trusted us." That was all he said.

The last thing that we were asked was to agree to turn off James's life support. My husband was adamant that the surgeon be involved in that decision. The surgeon did not make himself available, and he did not come back to the hospital. It required my husband's pushing the clinicians, the cardiologist, and social worker to call the surgeon. We had a phone consult in the PCICU and agreed as a team that nothing more could be done for James and that we would turn off the life support.

After the phone call, which was at 8:00 a.m. on Saturday, we were told that we could not stay in the PCICU, but that they would call when we could come and be with him. I interpreted that to mean that when they were ready to turn off the machines I would be able to be there and hold my son. Three hours passed and they called us and said that we could come down. When the PCICU doors opened this time I saw a bright light at his isolette and he was all swaddled up. He had not been swaddled before, ever. There were no machines attached and there were a couple of rocking chairs set up. The nurse pulled the drape around us and they told us we could hold him and stay as long as we wanted.

Somebody placed him in my arms and he was ice cold. I felt so bad, I could not look at him. I still apologize to him for that. My husband held him for a little bit and handed him back to me and a few minutes later I put him back in the isolette and we walked away. It was the last time I saw him. There were no social workers, no chaplain, nobody escorted us back to the room. We placed all that we had brought for our son, his blanket, and his outfit that he was going to wear home, into a wagon. We packed up our stuff and dragged the wagon through the hospital and brought it home.

Finding Answers

The day after James's funeral I handwrote a note to the hospital asking for anything that had his name on it. I wanted all his records. I wanted something of his that I could keep for the rest of my life.

We got a manila envelope back with five or six pages of lab values. After 11 days in the hospital and repeated surgeries, that was it!

I found an article about a mom with a baby boy who also had a coarctation of the aorta, who happened to be operated on by the same surgeon, and had had a bad outcome. I reached out to the authors of this article and asked to talk to the mother. They referred me to her attorney, who had been their source of information. The mother was not ready to talk to me, but the attorney was quite ready to offer his support and help me find answers. I was not looking for an attorney; I was looking for someone who understood how this could have happened. But finding the attorney turned out to be how we accomplished that. If I had not pursued litigation we would have never known any of what we now know.

On the day before what would have been James's fourth birthday, we received a call from our attorney. There had been a settlement offer of $750,000, to be accompanied by a gag order not to discuss the case. My counteroffer was to ask for fees, which my attorneys said were about $45,000 to $50,000 at that point, and a 5-minute conversation with the surgeon. The answer was no.

So we went to trial. We found out much that we had not known, like the fact that there had been a broken ventilator in surgery and the details of breakdown in handover communications between clinical teams. We found out that they had electively taken the breathing tube away from James as soon as we had left the PCICU that first afternoon after his original surgery. He had never breathed above the ventilator when they did that. They took blood gases every 10 to 15 minutes, but maybe nobody was reading them, because the trend was that the carbon dioxide was rising and the oxygen saturation levels were dropping. This downward spiral continued until his oxygen saturation was down into the 50s and his carbon dioxide was up into the 80s, when normal is 40–50. Then they gave him morphine, and 20 minutes after that he crashed. He cried out and somebody looked over and saw that he was gray. This was the "sudden, serious event" that had caused James's brain damage.

Although we were told that there was somebody with our son all the time during the hours that we were not allowed to be there with him, nobody was watching him closely. The doctor who was the attending physician had been called in to cover for another doctor. He had received a quick handoff and gone to get some dinner. The nurse practitioner was in the cafeteria. The bedside nurse was in the break room.

The jury found a verdict of neglect against the hospital clinicians, but they were not held responsible; my understanding is that the jury thought James's providers were negligent, but because of his heart defect did not think the negligence caused his death. After my attorney's mistrial motion was denied by the same judge who heard the case, I put on the brakes and told them that I had most of the answers to my questions and that I thought we could live with what we did not know. We did not want to pursue further legal action.

Conclusion

I went back to graduate school and got a master's in education in restorative practices, which is a conciliation method. I organized a community project called James's Project that engages in a range of projects to support newborn well-being, including patient advocacy programs for infant caregivers. We championed a bill that became law in 2014, requiring pulse oximetry screening in newborns in Pennsylvania. I wrote a book about James's story because it is a tough story to tell all the time, but also because I needed all the stakeholders who were involved to get a full picture of what really happened. My book is called *Split the Baby: One Child's Journey Through Medicine and Law* (Mannix, 2011). The title was not intended to be graphic, but actually quotes my attorney in the motion for a mistrial because he likened the jury's verdict to the Biblical story of

King Solomon who recommended splitting the baby under contention as a way to resolve a conflict.

In the course of writing the book, I reached out to most of the clinicians who were involved and learned more about James's case. For example, I reached out to the doctor who had come to our room and told us there was a sudden event, the same doctor who had gone out to dinner. He and I sat down and had a conversation in the middle of a hospital lobby and he told me that he had just completed a 24-hour shift when he was called in to cover for another physician. He feels that he failed his patient, our son and us. I feel that they and we failed our son. But I also have to take ownership of this failure and realize that this is part of my experience.

Case Discussion

In the early days of pediatric cardiac surgery, mortality rates were routinely above 50%. During the past three decades, survival among children born with even the most complex cardiac defects has increased substantially. By 2005–2009, discharge mortality for index cardiac operations reported to the Society of Thoracic Surgeons' congenital heart surgery database had fallen to 4.0% (Jacobs et al., 2011). Still, there is certainly no room for complacency. Mortality rates between institutions vary, indicating potential modifiable factors related to case volume, experience, and practice variability. Preventable adverse events may occur related to both technical and nontechnical factors associated with decision making, leadership, and management (Jacobs et al., 2008). Complications result in higher morbidity, long-term disability, decreased quality of life, and increased cost to the health system.

The field of pediatric cardiac care has received worldwide recognition as a leader in quality and patient safety and has advocated for system-wide changes in organizational culture. The field has many complex procedures that depend on a sophisticated organizational structure, the coordinated efforts of a team of individuals, and high levels of cognitive and technical performance (Galvan et al., 2005). In this regard, the field shares many properties with high-technology systems in which performance and outcomes depend on complex individual, technical, and organizational factors and the interactions among them. These shared properties include the specific context of complex team-based care, the acquisition and maintenance of individual skills, the role and reliance on technology, and the impact of working conditions on enabling great team performance.

Several factors have been linked to poor outcomes in pediatric cardiac care, including institutional and surgeon- or operator-specific volumes, case complexity, team coordination and collaboration, and systems failures (deLeval et al., 2000). Safety and organizational resilience in these organizations ultimately is understood as a characteristic of the system—the sum of all its parts plus their interactions. Interventions to improve quality and strategies to implement change should be directed to improve and reduce variations in outcomes. An obstacle to achieving these objectives is a lack of appreciation of the human factors in the field, including a poor understanding of the complexity of interactions between the technical task, the stresses of the treatment settings, the consequences of rigid staff hierarchies, the lack of time to brief and debrief, and cultural norms that resist change. Technical skills are fundamental to good outcomes, but nontechnical skills—coordination, cooperation, listening, negotiating, and so on—can also markedly influence the performance of individuals and teams and the outcomes of treatment (Schraagen et al., 2011). It is only through open communication and collaboration within and between organizations that we can foster excellence in clinical practice and innovation in pediatric cardiac surgical care.

In James's case, the system was clearly not designed for delivering reliable care. Some of what happened to James may have happened because clinicians lacked what has been called "psychological safety" and were afraid to speak up (Kennedy, 2001). This case also highlights the important role of patients and families. This case and others should stimulate discussion about the barriers that teams and organizations need to overcome and the changes that teams and organizations need to develop in order to engage families and deliver safe and resilient care.

Questions

1. The overarching theme in James's story is the absence of meaningful informed consent. At what points in James's diagnosis and treatment do you see the informed consent process breaking down? What do you think James's healthcare providers should have done differently to more effectively communicate with James's parents?

2. James's parents felt that they were not allowed to participate in their son's care and were excluded from key moments that would have allowed their baby to experience warmth and human contact. What policies do you think could be put in place to prevent this from happening? How do you think the absence of such policies might have affected James's care?

3. James's initial downturn came when he was not closely observed after being removed from the ventilator. This was apparently exacerbated by a poor handover process. What handover practices could be used to ensure effective communication of key information and oversight of patients?

4. James's parents were given little information about what had happened to their son, either while they were in the hospital or when they requested their son's records. This ultimately led to a protracted, costly legal battle. The parents say their legal course had only one purpose—to find out what had happened to their son. There are now programs that are designed to prevent this sort of adversarial outcome by responding openly and proactively to adverse events. How do you think the presence of such a program might help avoid unnecessary legal action and help healthcare providers learn from their mistakes?

5. Which of the core competencies for health professions are most relevant for this case? Why?

References

deLeval, M., Carthey, J., Wright, D. J., Farewell, V. T., & Reason, J. T. (2000). Human factors and cardiac surgery: A multicenter study. *Journal of Thoracic and Cardiovascular Surgery, 119*(4 Pt 1), 661–672.

Galvan, C., Bacha, E., Mohr, J., & Barach, P. (2005). A human factors approach to understanding patient safety during pediatric cardiac surgery. *Progress in Pediatric Cardiology, 20*(1), 13–20.

Gargiulo, G., Napoleone P., Angeli, E., & Oppido, G. (2008). Neonatal coarctation repair using extended end-to-end anastomosis. *Multimedia Manual Cardio-Thoracic Surgery, 328.*

Jacobs, J. P., Jacobs, M. L. Mavroudis, C., Backer, C. L., Lacour-Gayet, F. G., Tchervenkoy, C. I., . . . Edwards, F. H. (2008). Nomenclature and databases for the surgical treatment of congenital cardiac disease—an updated primer and an analysis of opportunities for improvement. *Cardiology in the Young, 18*(Suppl 2), 38–62.

Jacobs, J. P., O'Brien, S. M., Pasquali, S. K., Jacobs, M. L., Lacour-Gayet, F. G., Tchervenkov, C. I., . . Mavroudis, C. (2011). Variation in outcomes for benchmark operations: An analysis of the Society of Thoracic Surgeons Congenital Heart Surgery Database. *Annals of Thoracic Surgery, 92*(6), 2184–2191; discussion 2191–2192.

Kennedy, I. (2001). *Learning from Bristol: The report of the public inquiry into children's heart surgery at the Bristol Royal Infirmary 1984–1995.* London: Department of Health.

Mannix, M. E. (2011). *Split the baby: One child's journey through medicine and law.* Raleigh, NC: Lulu Press.

Matsui, H., & Gardiner, H. (2009). Coarctation of the aorta: Fetal and postnatal diagnosis and outcome: Anatomy of aortic coarctation: Lessons from the cardiac morphologists. *Medscape Pediatrics.* Available at: http://www.medscape.org/viewarticle/589271_2.

Rosenthal, E. (2005). Coarctation of the aorta from fetus to adult: Curable condition or life long disease process? *Heart, 91*(11), 1495–1502.

Schraagen, J. M., Schouten, T., Smit, M., Haas, F., van der Beek, D., van de Ven, J., & Barach P. (2011). A prospective study of paediatric cardiac surgical microsystems: Assessing the relationships between non-routine events, teamwork and patient outcomes. *BMJ Quality and Safety, 20*(7), 599–603.

Knowledge for Practice

Healthcare professionals must demonstrate knowledge of established and evolving biomedical, clinical, epidemiological, and social-behavioral sciences, and the application of this knowledge to patient care. Specific competencies within the Knowledge for Practice domain are to:

- Demonstrate an investigatory and analytic approach to clinical situations.
- Apply established and emerging scientific principles fundamental to health care for patients and populations.
- Apply established and emerging principles of clinical sciences to diagnostic and therapeutic decision making, clinical problem solving, and other aspects of evidence-based health care.
- Apply principles of epidemiological sciences to the identification of health problems, risk factors, treatment strategies, resources, and disease prevention/health promotion efforts for patients and populations.
- Apply principles of social-behavioral sciences to provision of patient care, including assessment of the impact of psychosocial and cultural influences on health, disease, care seeking, care compliance, and barriers to and attitudes toward care.

- Contribute to the creation, dissemination, application, and translation of new healthcare knowledge and practices.

The three cases presented in Section 2 represent patient harm in three very different areas: obstetrics, medication safety, and missed diagnosis. As in other sections of the book, we caution the reader that these cases are complex and include elements of other competencies as well. As you read the cases, it is helpful to think about the other competencies that are relevant. (Refer to the full list of competencies in the appendix.)

Case 5, "I'm Left in Fear: An Account of Harm in Maternity Care," tells the story of "Amelia," a native of Africa who was living in the United Kingdom. Amelia's first child had been born by cesarean section, and she had made an informed decision to try for a vaginal birth with her second child. Due to a series of miscalculations, Amelia suffered a uterine rupture, stillbirth, and massive blood loss.

Case 6, "A Routine Endoscopic Procedure," is about Dorothy Johnson who, in 2006, had an endoscopic retrograde cholangiopancreatography (ERCP) and a sphincterotomy in an outpatient clinic. Dorothy's daughters, Anetta Parker and Dorothy Johnson Prince, discuss the events leading to their mother's death from what they had assumed to be a simple outpatient procedure.

Case 7, "The Last Run: An Undiagnosed Heart Rhythm Disturbance," is about Alex James, a 19-year-old university student in the United States. Alex's father, James, tells the story of Alex's fatal heart arrhythmia that was not recognized and diagnosed.

I'm Left in Fear: An Account of Harm in Maternity Care

The Story of Amelia (United Kingdom)

Nicola Mackintosh, Kylie Watson, Susanna Rance, and Jane Sandall

"This is what my midwife was telling me at every antenatal clinic. 'If you go into labor you are supposed to come over to the hospital because you need to be monitored.'"

Editors' Note

Amelia is a 38-year-old woman from Africa living in the United Kingdom (UK). In 2008, Amelia's first child was delivered in the hospital by an uneventful elective cesarean section. When Amelia became pregnant again in 2009, health professionals informed her she could have a vaginal birth after cesarean section (VBAC). 72 to 76% of women are able to have a successful vaginal birth after a single previous cesarean birth (RCOG, 2007). Women need to be well informed about both the benefits and the potential harm of a planned VBAC (Horey, Weaver, & Russell, 2004). One uncommon, but potentially serious, complication associated with a previous cesarean is a ruptured uterus, where the previous cesarean scar breaks down. This can occur before the start of labor or, more commonly, during labor. This complication can be life-threatening for both the woman and the baby. The incidence of uterine rupture for women attempting a trial of labor after a previous cesarean section is 22–74 of every 10,000 women (RCOG, 2007). The signs of uterine rupture can include bleeding, pain, and the baby showing signs of distress in labor.

LEARNING OBJECTIVES

After completing this case study, you will be able to:

1. Describe the challenges patients face in trying to be heard by health-care professionals.

2. Discuss an appropriate organizational response to systematic failure to care.

3. Explore the growing partnership model in which patients are treated as equal partners in decision making about their care.

Amelia's Story

Amelia presented late in her first pregnancy (at 8 months) to her local hospital. The maternity staff informed her that she needed an elective cesarean section because of a medical condition. Amelia describes being happy with this decision, and she had faith that the staff were acting in her best interests: "I was with the right people, so I knew they were doing the right thing for me. I trusted them."

In 2009, Amelia became pregnant again. Because of her underlying medical condition, she was looked after by a specialist team of community midwives who provided continuity of care during her pregnancy. Her midwife offered Amelia the choice to deliver vaginally, but explained the risk of scar rupture. According to Amelia:

When I saw the midwife when I was pregnant she asked, "Do you want to go for normal birth or do you want a cesarean?" And I was shocked, I was like, "Can someone who [has had] a cesarean go for a normal birth?" She said, "Yeah! Hundreds of the women are coming here and they are giving birth [normally], but the moment you go into labor, you have to come to the hospital, you need to be monitored . . . if we see the scar is opening we have to rush you to the operating theater, we have to remove the baby, to protect you and the baby."

Amelia made an informed choice and agreed with her care givers to try for a vaginal birth. Her pregnancy was uneventful, and she describes feeling well throughout the 9-month pregnancy. She reports receiving excellent care from her specialist team, and she was booked to deliver at her local hospital. Amelia was seen at the hospital antenatal clinic and had an ultrasound scan nine days after her due date, The scan showed her baby was healthy.

The following evening a Saturday, Amelia started to experience mild contractions. By Sunday morning she called the hospital staff and told them she was in labor. The specialist team of midwives that had looked after Amelia throughout her pregnancy was not available during the weekend, but they had given her a number to call and assured her that staff would know what care she needed. She called the on-call community midwife and was told not to go to the hospital yet as her contractions were 30 minutes apart. Because her contractions were not too strong, Amelia was happy with this advice, and her partner supported her decision. She went to her partner's house, they had supper together, and she tried to sleep. At 3:00 a.m. Monday morning the contractions suddenly became stronger. After having a bath, Amelia noticed that she was bleeding, so her partner called an ambulance. Despite being told that she was overdue, bleeding, and had a scar that needed monitoring, the ambulance staff requested that Amelia ring the midwife so that they could authorize her transfer. When Amelia rang the community on-call team, the midwife told her "not to worry" and tried to persuade her to take a bath and wait before coming in. However, Amelia was insistent:

Look, I've told you I'm in pain and when the pain comes I feel like pushing, understand? And I was told that the moment I go into labor I should come to the hospital, because I need to be monitored.

The midwife agreed that she could come in via ambulance and said she would notify the labor ward that she was on her way. Amelia left her older son with her partner and was taken to the hospital early Monday morning alone: "I wasn't expecting [problems], I didn't think that I needed to go with somebody, I was going to the people I trusted, I knew I was going to get good care."

When Amelia arrived on the labor ward, the ambulance staff gave her maternity records to the receptionist and handed over her details. Amelia was told to wait in the reception area until a midwife was available to take her into the labor ward. There were two other women waiting in the reception area with Amelia, and no chairs were free so Amelia ended up sitting on the floor. As Amelia waited, her pain started to intensify, and she became progressively more distressed. Her presenting history, including her medical condition and her previous cesarean section, were not taken into account despite her insistence that she needed immediate attention.

I waited. I was in pain. Someone was on the chair. I'm on the floor. So . . . after some time . . . I'm sitting down, I can't see anybody, I saw on the clock it was another hour [and] nobody has come to see me. I stood up, I talked to the receptionist. I told her, "Look, I was brought here by ambulance, I'm in pain, I'm overdue, and I have a scar which needs monitoring." She told me, "You see those two ladies there? They came before you." I went back and I sat, but I was in pain. The ladies who were sitting there they were not in pain. They were heavily pregnant but they were not in pain, they were sitting with their partners, while I was down on the floor. I stayed there.

Amelia was anxious to be seen by a member of the clinical staff, believing that once they read her records, they would appreciate the urgency of monitoring her condition:

The receptionist is not medically trained. But she would have known somebody . . . who is trained, [who could] come and see me. I think if someone had read my file they would have said, "I think this lady needs to be monitored, she needs to be cared for, somebody has to be there for her." Not just to be left alone on my own, in the reception room.

Amelia had the sense that she needed to "fight" her way into the labor ward to be seen by clinical staff. Yet she did not want to create trouble for herself by offending the hospital staff so she complied with the instructions given by the receptionist and continued to wait:

Maybe if I was arrogant . . . I would have made things worse. There's no way I could have forced myself inside. I said, "I've been brought in by an ambulance . . ." I told her what needs to be done on me, she's just telling me those two ladies come before you, which I didn't understand. I stayed there. I said OK. I think fine, I'm in the hospital, OK, I'll deal with it. I stayed there with my pain for 2 and a half hours.

The night that Amelia was admitted was busy with double the usual number of admissions. When Amelia was admitted onto the labor ward more than 2 hours after first arriving, she was assigned to the midwife who was the shift coordinator who was also responsible for managing the labor ward for the shift. Because there were no spare delivery rooms, Amelia was put in a "prep room," which was a small room where women were prepared for the operating theater. Delivery rooms were normally equipped with cylinders of pain relieving gas (Entonox), and cardiotocograph (CTG) monitors, which assess the baby's well-being and uterine contractions. In this prep room, there was no Entonox, and the CTG monitor was fixed to the wall, which limited the ability to monitor women on the bed.

[The midwife] took me inside. Then she asked me, "What has brought you here?" I said, "Please, I'm in labor. I'm overdue, I have a scar which needs monitoring." Then she said, "OK, sit there." I sat down on the bed. Then she said, "OK, we need to monitor the baby." So she put a monitor on and she told me to hold it. She said, "I have to go and look for the belt." When she went to look for the belt she stayed away for 30 minutes. I couldn't hold the monitor anymore because the pain. I had to go on the floor, at least when the pain comes I could hold [on to] something [the bed], because of the pain I couldn't hold the monitor anymore.

When the midwife coordinator came back, she examined Amelia and said she was 8 cm dilated and should be transferred to another room ready for the delivery. She left again saying that she would be back. However, she did not come back. Amelia described the anguish of being left alone in pain. She tried to call the attention of staff who were getting ready to start the next shift, but no one came to help her.

She left me alone in the room. I'm in pain. I'm pushing. I don't know what is happening. I'm just on my own, I'm screaming, I'm calling everybody's name, I remember I crawled, I opened the door. I saw a lady and a gentleman standing in the corridor putting on their uniform, and I say, "Please, come and help me, I'm giving birth to my baby." Then the lady said, "OK, let me come see you." Then she come and peeped in the room, then said, "Ah! Someone is going to come and help you, go back." I had to go back in the room, I stayed alone . . . I think for almost an hour.

Because the shift was so busy, the whiteboard that was used to record details about every admission had not been updated, and details of Amelia's medical history were not there. They were also omitted from the handover at the start of the next shift. When a new midwife came into Amelia's room on the morning shift to take over her care, the midwife presumed that this was Amelia's first baby. Further delays were incurred while the new midwife went to find an Entonox cylinder and monitoring equipment.

By this stage, Amelia described herself as very weak and the pain level was "too much." She had started vomiting. She said she felt that she was dying and was desperate for the staff to make her pain go away. As the midwife tried to move Amelia to a laboring room it became clear that she was seriously ill. She then lost consciousness.

They are trying to put me on the commode and take me to the bathtub. I'm telling them, "Please, I'm dying." As they are lifting me, they are saying, "Can you help us? I mean . . . put your leg up." I said, "I can't, because I'm weak, help me." I felt I can't do any more . . . I collapsed. That's when they realized that things have gone wrong. I could hear people moving around . . . I heard someone coming in and saying, "Oh this lady is in danger." The only thing I could hear [were] people . . . rushing around, that was it.

Emergency help was called, and the new midwife coordinator and consultant obstetrician arrived to assist. A scan revealed there was no fetal heartbeat and her abdomen was full of blood. Amelia was taken to the operating theatre immediately. There was 3.5 liters of blood in her abdomen. Amelia suffered a rupture of her uterus, stillbirth, and massive blood loss (4 liters of blood in total). She was hypotensive and critically ill and had to be transferred to the intensive care unit for resuscitation.

The Consequences for Amelia

After her surgery, Amelia spoke to senior doctors and some midwives on a number of different occasions about the events leading up to her collapse. One of the consultants admitted that the hospital had failed her:

I saw the doctor who worked on me, who told me, "Oh Amelia you were very, very sick, you almost lost your life." And she told me, "We really have no . . . answers to your questions. We failed to care for you."

The maternity unit rarely closed its doors to admissions because of a desire to keep the service running for the local community. A midwife told Amelia that on the night she was admitted the labor ward had been unusually busy. Amelia expressed anger in the interview that "busy-ness" was somehow used to excuse what happened to her and the death of her baby:

She was telling me, "The hospital was busy, you know." I couldn't understand it; even if the hospital is busy I don't think someone deserves to die. This is not a Third World country, like in Africa where you can't go to the hospital. There you tell them, "I'm contracting," they tell you to go back home. You give birth under a tree.

Amelia reported feeling shocked and traumatized by the organization's lack of care and compassion when she kept asking for help. She contrasted this with the caring relationships she had with her general practitioner and the specialist midwifery team who had cared for her antenatally.

I try to figure out the hearts of the people who are in the hospital. I really don't see how someone can come in and see a patient who is in pain and really don't care. You show that you don't care. [For] 9 months I was pregnant but [for] only a few hours, someone doesn't even care.

Amelia's trust in the healthcare system and staff working within it was broken. She lost trust in the system. She was left to believe that patients needed to have someone with them in order to receive safe care.

I've gone to the hospital, knowing I've gone for help, I didn't even bother going with anybody. Now [if] I'm going to the hospital, I have to go with somebody. I don't trust them anymore, which I just find awful. Even the people who are qualified do their jobs, I . . . I don't trust them, even if I go to the GP [general practitioner] . . . I don't think he's going to do the right thing on me. I'm just left . . . with no trust in people, I'm left in fear.

Amelia also wondered whether she could have done more to make herself heard and described being left with feelings of guilt.

This is what I'm asking myself. Didn't I look [like] someone who is in pain? Did the receptionist want some money from me? I don't know. I just ask questions myself and I have to answer them . . . by myself. Maybe I would have used force to enter [the labor ward] but it is the same midwives on the phone, inside there, the one who left me in the room . . . so what was I supposed to do? Was I supposed to tell the ambulance, "Look, don't leave me here, take me to another hospital?" I keep on maybe blaming myself, where did I go wrong? I went in to hospital at the right time and I think I went to the right people, thinking I was going to be helped.

Two years later, Amelia was still receiving psychological counseling about the incident.

Conclusion

Amelia shared her story regarding the complications women experience during childbirth. Amelia's account provides a powerful illustration of the interlinked contribution of system-level processes that can contribute to patient safety incidents and harm, and Amelia was very keen for lessons to be learned from her story.

Case Discussion

Amelia's case highlights the difficulties faced by patients trying to ensure their own safety and well-being and, in Amelia's case, that of her baby. Amelia was well informed about the risks of pursuing a VBAC (Horey et al., 2004), and at various stages in her labor she alerted staff that she needed monitoring and close supervision. On numerous occasions, in spite of her prodding, the providers and the organization failed to respond promptly and appropriately. They dismissed her concerns and neglected to attend to her needs.

A range of system issues aligned in Amelia's case to create many lost opportunities and delays (Reason, 2000). First, there was a lack of continuity of care. Amelia's midwife, who had provided care throughout pregnancy and provided her with advice regarding what should happen during her labor, was off duty and another midwife on-call advised her on admission. This resulted in delays, confusion, and lack of continuity of care. Furthermore, it was a weekend where complications are known to be more frequent due to less supervision and less senior providers on shift.

The admitting unit was extremely busy, staff had become used to workarounds to cope with the heavy patient workload, and the practices had drifted beyond the boundaries of safe operation (Amalberti, Vincent, Auroy, & de Saint Maurice, 2006). Amelia was not triaged by a clinician on admission, resulting in further delays. She was admitted to a room where essential monitoring equipment was missing, resulting in further delays. Her details were not recorded on the whiteboard, and there was no handover at shift change regarding her high risk history nor her protestations about her pain and escalating complaints.

This tragic case highlights the importance of an organization's response during and after an incident. Amelia reported being profoundly affected, both physically and psychologically, by the lack of care and compassion shown to her during her labor and in the aftermath of the adverse event (Beck, 2004, 2006).

Questions

1. How many times did Amelia have to speak up and insist that her and her baby's health was at risk? What was the response on each occasion? Why do you think she was met with this response?

2. What might the system failures have been in Amelia's care in relation to each of the following:

   a. Transfer and admission to the labor ward

   b. Out-of-hours service provision

    c. Assessment and triage

    d. Communication and handover process

    e. Staffing and management of the labor ward

    f. Facilities and equipment

    g. Managing the adverse event, including full disclosure and patient support

3. How could the organization have helped demonstrate to Amelia that the lessons from her tragic case were being attended to and polices had changed after the event?

4. What are your feelings about the woman's account of the events?

5. What are potential strategies to address the needs of a culturally and linguistically diverse patient population? Do you think minorities have difficulty with ensuring their concerns are taken seriously and in timely manner?

6. Which of the core competencies for health professions do you think are most relevant for this case? Why?

References

Amalberti, R., Vincent, C., Auroy, Y., & de Saint Maurice, G. (2006). Violations and migrations in health care: A framework for understanding and management. *Quality and Safety in Health Care, 15*(Suppl 1), i66–i71.

Beck, C. T. (2004). Birth trauma: In the eye of the beholder. *Nursing Research, 53*(1), 28–35.

Beck, C. T. (2006). Pentadic cartography: Mapping birth trauma narratives. *Qualitative Health Research, 16*(4), 453–466.

Horey, D., Weaver, J., & Russell, H. (2004). Information for pregnant women about caesarean birth (Review). *Cochrane Database Systematic Reviews*. DOI: 10.1002/14651858.CD003858.pub2

RCOG. (2007). *Birth after previous caesarean section: RCOG green-top guideline no 45*. London: RCOG Press.

Reason, J. (2000). Human error: Models and management. *BMJ, 320*(7237), 768–770.

A Routine Endoscopic Procedure

The Story of Dorothy Johnson (United States)

Julie Johnson, Helen Haskell, and Paul Barach

Editors' Note

Dorothy Johnson was the matriarch of a large, close-knit family. Her husband died when she was only 45, leaving her with nine children, one of whom also died young. Mrs. Johnson was closely involved in the lives of her surviving eight children and her many grandchildren. A religious woman, she busied herself in church and community and provided spiritual guidance and support to her children and others. At age 74, she was vigorous and independent.

In December 2006, Mrs. Johnson's daughter Anetta drove her to an endoscopy clinic for an outpatient procedure known as endoscopic retrograde cholangiopancreatography (ERCP). Mrs. Johnson underwent a sphincterotomy as part of her procedure. In a series of interviews with the editors, Dorothy's daughters Anetta Parker and Dorothy Prince reflected upon the death of their mother following what they thought was a simple out-patient procedure.

LEARNING OBJECTIVES

After completing this case study, you will be able to:

1. Discuss the implications of medical and procedural overtreatment.
2. Compare the relative safety of procedures performed in the hospital versus ambulatory clinics.

3. Discuss the importance of authentic and timely communication with patients and families.

4. Assess the impact of integrated healthcare systems on cost-effective and safe care.

A Routine Endoscopic Procedure

Our mother usually had an endoscopic procedure every 2 years. We thought that she had too many visits with her gastroenterologist. She saw the gastroenterologist about every 30 or 60 days. When we asked the physician why our mother had to come in on a continuous basis, his response was "acid reflux." She was taking a proton pump inhibitor for her acid reflux.

Our mother had an endoscopy of her upper gastrointestinal tract in September 2006. The gastroenterologist wanted her to come back in December for another endoscopic test. We did not think it was a good idea for her to have two tests so close together, but she made her own decisions, and she wanted to follow what the doctor recommended. We took her to the endoscopy unit at the hospital for an ERCP on December 12, 2006. An hour and a half after the procedure began the doctor came out and told us that the ERCP procedure was done and that everything looked good. He said, however, that he had to cut her bile duct to relieve the pressure in the biliary tree. We later learned that this was called a sphincterotomy. He said that everything should be okay and to bring her back in 2 weeks. He told us to give her Tylenol for pain.

Mom began regurgitating everything she drank. She was perspiring and was in pain. I called the hospital and told the nurse to get the doctor. The nurse replied that the doctor was unavailable and to give her Tylenol. I told the nurse that she did not understand, that on a pain tolerance scale from 1 to 10 my mother's pain was at a 9. The nurse kept saying to continue to give her Tylenol—but Mom could not keep the Tylenol down.

The physician called back about 5 minutes later and said to try to give her one Tylenol and some soup. I told him that she was regurgitating and that she could not hold anything down. I told him we needed to bring her back to the hospital and asked that he make her a direct admission so we would not have to wait in the emergency room.

Upon arriving at the emergency room we discovered that the doctor had not made her a direct admission. They did not know she was coming. The doctor had turned off his cell phone as he was no longer on call, and he had not given a report to his on-call colleague. This meant that the emergency room had no knowledge of our mom's condition nor that we were bringing her in.

A 12-Hour Wait

Our mother moaned and was in great pain in the emergency room. We had never heard her moan before. Dorothy went out to the parking lot and called the doctor from her cell phone. But it was after 5:00 p.m. and he didn't pick up. The answering service called the doctor's colleague, who said that she couldn't do anything because Mom's doctor would have to be the one to give the orders. But the emergency room never received any orders from him. They did the full workup for abdominal pain, and it took over 12 hours before she even got any pain medication.

The emergency department sent her to her hospital room at maybe 5:00 or 6:00 a.m. the next morning. At 5:00 p.m. that evening, Mother was still vomiting. That was 24 hours of vomiting, and her doctor still hadn't been to see her. About 9:00 p.m. Mom started going downhill. Her breathing changed. She was struggling for air. Dorothy spoke to the nurse at the desk, who said, "We can't just give your mother oxygen. We have to get it okayed by the doctor."

Dorothy was experienced as a medical assistant and she knew what to ask. She said, "Okay, can you give the doctor a call?"

Even so, we did not get the okay until 11:00 or 12:00 p.m. that night. By that time, Mother couldn't urinate any more, either. The next morning they came and put in a catheter. After they put the catheter in, they elected to move her up to medical ICU. We never knew who gave these orders. No doctor had been to see her.

She stayed in the medical ICU maybe 3 hours. While she was there they put in a central venous line, and then she was moved to the critical care intensive care unit (CCU). We don't know who gave the orders for that, either. So within 24 hours of admission she was moved from the emergency room to the ward, to the ICU, and then to the CCU. At this time her bloodwork showed that her kidneys were shutting down. Her lungs were filling up with fluid, her pancreas was messed up, and her diabetes was out of control. She just kept spiraling down. They said she had sepsis.

Code Blue

Now that Mom was in ICU, she had a pulmonologist and a kidney doctor, and her gastroenterologist's two colleagues had also come to see her and looked at the chart. But we still had not heard from the physician who performed the procedure. On the third day of admission, on Friday, December 15, we took our oldest brother and walked over to the physician's office just before closing time. We asked to speak to the doctor and we sat and waited. We asked him what he had done and what had gone wrong. He drew a little picture of the stomach and esophagus and said that one of her bile ducts had been clotted and he had slit it to allow it to drain. He said that inflammation of the pancreas was to be expected after this operation.

That evening, after the visit to the doctor's office, my husband took me out to a movie to try to get me away from the hospital. But as soon as I sat in my seat my cell phone went off. It was my 12-year-old son calling from the hospital, and he said that something was wrong with Grandma. It was approximately 10:00 p.m. on December 15.

I called the nurses' station, gave them my name, and asked if something was wrong with my mother. They said yes, there was a resuscitation code in my mom's room. I immediately rushed to the hospital and ran up to my mom's room.

A nurse came out and told us that she needed someone to go into our mother's room and speak to her to see if she was coherent. They had revived her, but because she had lost oxygen for so long they needed to know if her brain was okay. So I walked into my mom's room and I whispered into her ear. I grabbed her hand and placed my other hand on her forehead and I began to speak to her. I said, "Mom, this is Anetta. If you recognize my voice, I need you to squeeze my hand"—and she did. I told my mom that I loved her and I quoted her a prayer of faith. I told her that I believed there would be a miraculous healing that night.

The Final Days

The next day, December 16, Mom's original doctor finally came to see her. By this time she had pneumonia and sepsis and had been placed on a ventilator. The doctor assessed Mom's stomach, which was very swollen, and said that all the necessary specialists had been assigned. He was still saying that pancreatitis after ERCP was common and that he was optimistic she would get well.

Although she was on a ventilator, Mom was very coherent. She wrote us notes, telling us different things she wanted us to do. She always wanted her back rubbed, and she would want us to bathe her a second time after the nurses had bathed her. Dorothy stayed in the hospital the entire time, and she was very involved in Mom's care. She read the progress notes in Mom's chart and made suggestions. She asked them to explain her lab values and gave them a list of her meds. She never left except to get a change of clothes.

On December 27, about 4:00 a.m., as Mom was having a bath she had a cardiac arrest and was coded. Dorothy had gone home to change clothes. The nurse was supposed to call, but she did not. When we arrived and asked the nurse what had happened, she said that when she was suctioning our mom she felt some resistance. She continued to try and suction her as she coded.

Dorothy rushed into the room. She was determined to be by Mother's side. They worked on Mom for about 25 to 30 minutes but they were not able to revive her. Finally the doctor declared her death. That was it.

Raising Awareness

After Mom's death, I knew we had to do something. I sent certified letters to the Texas Medical Board, the Texas Department of State Health Services, The Joint Commission, the director of the emergency room, and the new CEO of the hospital, along with the physician who had done the procedure. I sent the letters to everyone I thought could give me answers and raise awareness in regards to our mother's death. When you bring a patient back to the emergency room from a day procedure, somebody should be ready to take verbal or written orders so that no patient should have to sit in the emergency room for 12 hours.

The CEO of the hospital called me back about a month after Mother died. The hospital was under new management at this time. The new CEO set up a meeting for us with the physician and the CEO to explain what happened to our mom, but the physician declined to come. After a year the hospital sent another letter stating that the physician would now meet with the family. So we finally met with the physician. He told us that he was justified in having done the procedure on our mother, and that without an autopsy there was no way of knowing whether she had died as a result of the procedure or not. We were shocked at this comment. Our oldest sister had been asked privately about an autopsy when Mother died, but had declined. We did not know this would turn out to be so important.

We were very concerned and were not getting answers to our questions about what happened during the procedure and in the hospital. We decided to seek legal assistance to get the truth. We went through about 10 attorneys seeking to file a lawsuit against the physician, the hospital, and the emergency room for the neglect of our mother. And the doctor was right; without an autopsy most attorneys did not want to take a chance on the case. We finally found an attorney and were just 2 weeks short of the 2-year statute of limitations for filing a case with the court when our expert witness backed out and said he could not say without a shadow of a doubt that cutting the bile duct of my mother was negligent. So in the end we had no case to seek legal redress.

We filed a complaint with the Texas Medical Board. At first they found the doctor not negligent, but we won the right to appeal, and I went to Austin and sat in front of 20 board members and physicians of the Texas Medical Board. A year later they again found that the physician had acted within the standard of care in Texas.

Our decision to pursue legal and regulatory action was never about the money. As a family, we wanted the physician to apologize and say he could have done something different. He never acknowledged this.

The Department of Health Services did tell us that the emergency room was cited for the care that was given to my mother on that night, but they said the details were not available to the family. We felt that we should be able to see that information. Due to the laws of our state we were not allowed to have all the information that we wanted and needed to gain an understanding of the events that led to our mother's death.

Conclusion

Our mother liked her physician and cared for him, but everything that happened to her was directly related to the complications due to his care. Mom did not walk in on December 12 with pancreatitis, she did not walk in with fluid on her lungs, and she did not walk in with pneumonia or kidney failure. This all happened due to the procedure. After extensive research we found that this is what happens when the bile duct leaks into the body: it poisons the body.

Could there have been something that the physician could have done to prevent this from occurring?

I would advise patients and families to make sure that before any test or procedure there needs to be effective and honest communication with the doctor. I think that is what really needs to take place between a doctor and the patient and the patient's family. The doctor needs to talk about the eventual consequences.

Case Discussion

This is a difficult case to analyze because it isn't clear what happened to Dorothy Johnson, other than that there were a series of system failures. From her daughters' account, there were issues with communication with the doctor who performed the procedure. Mrs. Johnson's family felt abandoned by her doctor and felt that a primary factor in her death was the doctor's failure to follow up when their mother suffered complications from a procedure he had performed. This eventually led to their going to great lengths to file a lawsuit and to bring the doctor before the medical board. Anetta Parker subsequently wrote a book, *God's Grace Is Sufficient* (2011), in which she chronicled her thoughts and the family's thoughts throughout these experiences.

ERCP is a method of inspecting the ducts around the gallbladder and pancreas using an endoscope threaded through the mouth until it reaches the ampulla of Vater, a small opening where the pancreatic and bile ducts enter the duodenum. Dye is injected into the ducts to look for stones or other abnormalities, which can often be treated immediately by passing instruments through the endoscope. The most common intervention associated with ERCP is biliary sphincterotomy (Cotton & Leung, 2006). This involves cutting the sphincter muscle surrounding the ampulla of Vater and is usually done to improve bile drainage or to aid in the removal of bile stones. Complications of ERCP occur in approximately 5–10% of patients and can be serious, especially if infection is involved. Pancreatitis, the most frequent complication, occurs in about 5% of patients who undergo the procedure (Donnellan & Byrd, 2012). About 1% of

ERCP patients suffer serious long-term morbidity or death as a result of pancreatitis or perforation (Cotton & Leung, 2006).

Dr. Peter Cotton, one of the pioneers of ERCP procedures, believes that the technique is now widely overused. Overuse, particularly of diagnostic procedures, is considered to be a significant problem in health care, adding both to the cost of health care and to the burden of medical harm to patients (Cassels & Guest, 2012). Safe, noninvasive imaging techniques now produce images of equal quality to ERCP. The American College of Gastrointestinal Endoscopy and the National Institutes of Health recommend that ERCP be performed only for therapeutic, not diagnostic, purposes (National Institutes of Health, 2002). Nevertheless, overuse of ERCP and sphincterotomy is an ongoing controversy in the gastroenterological community. Studies of lawsuits suggest that ERCP is often done for diagnostic purposes for which it is not recommended and that it is frequently done by physicians who lack sufficient training and experience both in performing the procedure and in handling the ensuing complications (Cotton, 2010, 2011).

Dorothy Johnson underwent ERCP for reasons that are not entirely clear, but which almost certainly fell under the category of diagnostic rather than therapeutic, because she apparently had no explicit complaint and did not suffer from gallstones. The dictated summary of the procedure says that she was "troubled by recurrent epigastric abdominal discomfort." Following the procedure, she suffered many of the potential adverse effects of ERCP and sphincterotomy, including rapidly progressing pancreatitis, possibly complicated by duodenal perforation. Her condition was exacerbated by an extended wait in an emergency room that cost multiple hours at the beginning of her downward course and may have ultimately contributed to her deterioration in the hospital and her untimely death.

Questions

1. What were the system failures in Dorothy Johnson's care?
2. What is the physician's responsibility to follow up with a patient, and how do you think the reality differs from the

ideal? What can healthcare professionals do to make the follow-up process go more smoothly?

3. According to her daughters, even though Mrs. Johnson consented to the ERCP procedure, she did not know or did not understand that the doctor was going to perform a sphincterotomy. In Mrs. Johnson's case, the sphincterotomy was a nonemergency elective procedure. What does this say about the informed consent process in this case, and how do you think it could have been handled differently?

4. How do you think the problem of overuse of procedures such as ERCP can be addressed?

5. What should healthcare professionals do to communicate with patients following an adverse event? How can hospitals and clinics ensure that there is learning from these events?

6. What can we learn from this case about designing strategies to improve communication with patients and families who are undergoing a medical emergency?

7. Which of the core competencies for health professions are most relevant for this case? Why?

References

Cassels, C. K., & Guest, J. A. (2012). Choosing wisely: Helping physicians and patients make smart decisions about their care. *JAMA, 307*(17), 1801–1802.

Cotton, P. B. (2010). Twenty more ERCP lawsuits: Why? Poor indications and communications. *Gastrointestinal Endoscopy, 72*(4):904.

Cotton, P. B. (2011). Are low-volume ERCPists a problem in the United States? A plea to examine and improve ERCP practice—NOW. *Gastroenterological Endoscopy, 74*(1), 161–166.

Cotton, P.B., & Leung, J. W. (Eds.). (2006). *Advanced digestive endoscopy: ERCP*. Malden, MA: Blackwell Publishing.

Donnellan, F., & Byrd, M. F. (2012). Prevention of post-ERCP pancreatitis. *Gastroenterology Research and Practice*, Article ID 796751.

National Institutes of Health. (2002). Endoscopic retrograde cholangiopancreatography (ERCP) for diagnosis and therapy. State-of-the-Science Conference Statement, January 14–16. Available at: http://consensus.nih.gov/2002/2002ERCPsos020html.htm

Parker, A. (2011). *God's grace is sufficient: My personal journey from heartache to hope*. Mustang, OK: Tate Publishing.

The Last Run: An Undiagnosed Heart Rhythm Disturbance

The Story of Alex James (United States)

John James

Editors' Note

Nineteen-year-old Alex James was an Air Force officer-in-training with big ambitions. He attended military camps and pushed himself hard as a runner. But at the beginning of his junior year in college, this healthy, athletic young man collapsed while running in the Texas heat. Alex recovered without assistance and was taken to the hospital for evaluation. Three weeks after his release from the hospital he went for another run, collapsed again, and died. This account by Alex's father John reflects the events that transpired around the two incidents, and the reasons why John thinks Alex's ultimately fatal condition was not recognized.

LEARNING OBJECTIVES

After completing this case study, you will be able to:

1. Recognize the importance of diagnostic accuracy when using medical tests.

2. Demonstrate the importance of using evidence-based guidelines for the care of patients.

3. Outline ways of improving communication with patients and their families.

4. Discuss the issue of meaningful and transparent informed consent.

5. Illustrate ways of helping patients manage their underlying illness after being discharged from healthcare settings.

A Joyful Child

Alex was our firstborn son, and he was a delight. He was a smart kid, curious and very joyful as a child. He was a good student in high school, and when he went off to college he decided that he was going to be the best that he could be. I asked him the last week of his life what he wanted most of all, and he answered that he wanted to be an Air Force officer.

Alex was a passionate exerciser and runner. At the time of these events he was nearly 20 years old. He had been to summer camp in the military earlier in the summer. He was determined to make a perfect score on the Air Force physical fitness test, which is not easy. He came back home to Houston and continued to run in Houston in the summer. Houston in the summer is very hot and humid, a very difficult place to run. He and I ran a race late in July called the Lunar Rendezvous Run. That is the last race either of us ran.

Alex's Last Days

In mid-August, Alex returned to college. One evening he went running and collapsed. He recovered without assistance, but was taken by ambulance to the hospital. We were called at our home in Houston. I went up and stayed with Alex for 5 days while he was in the hospital. He was given a couple of electrocardiograms (ECGs) and the usual blood draw of electrolytes, glucose, etc. He had an echocardiogram and an exercise stress text, which he passed with flying colors.

He was under the care of a cardiologist. I mentioned to this doctor that I could go get an electrocardiogram that my son had had from the Air Force 6 months earlier. He said he was not interested. I was a little surprised, because the agency where I work actually has me carry a card with my baseline ECG on it. I was a little uneasy after this, but we really did not have much choice. Alex was in the hospital and being evaluated.

They told us that everything was normal, but then a consultant was called in. He recommended that Alex have a cardiac MRI scan and then possibly go on to have a heart catheterization, depending on the results. We were told afterward that the MRI did not show what they had hoped, so Alex then underwent a cardiac catheterization, which was done by the original admitting cardiologist. The catheterization showed nothing abnormal.

Of course, Alex had to give his informed consent for the heart cath. It was very traumatic for a 19-year-old boy. He was basically giving his doctors permission to open up his chest if anything should go wrong. But the doctor told us a story of a famous basketball player who had collapsed and died suddenly on the basketball court at the age of 40. This put a lot of fear in my son and in my wife and me as well. He signed the forms and we did not try to stop him. My son was so frightened that he could not write on the informed consent form. The nurse wrote for him and then he scrawled his signature at the bottom.

After the cardiac catheterization, I sat with Alex as we waited for the time to elapse before he was allowed to go home. He had a very painful groin hematoma and I remember him screaming. He had a huge lump on his groin. The nurse repacked his groin area to compress the hematoma.

He was discharged that evening with the understanding that he would go to another hospital the next morning for an electrophysiology test, a different kind of cardiac catheterization that was meant to check his heart rhythm. The electrophysiology test was done by a colleague of the first consultant. Once it was over I was invited in. The electrophysiologist said they could not find anything wrong. He recommended three things: one, that my son should not run until they sorted out some things; two, that they do some genetic testing at a major medical center; and three, that Alex should consider having a loop monitor inserted. He also suggested that Alex have a follow-up office visit with another physician 5 days later. I assumed that physician would be a cardiologist, but she turned out to be a physician-in-training in family medicine.

After the electrophysiology test, Alex was supposed to spend the day resting quietly in a hospital bed. At one point he got up briefly and the cut in his groin opened up and bled all over the place. That was really traumatic for him. They stopped the bleeding, mopped up the blood, and put him back in bed until late evening, when they finally discharged him.

Alex's discharge instructions said, "Don't drive for 24 hours." That was it. So he didn't drive for 24 hours. We went to a Mexican restaurant and talked about what they had offered him, which was a loop monitor to record abnormal heart rhythms. The loop monitor had to be activated by the patient if the patient experienced symptoms he thought should be recorded. We decided that would not be particularly helpful and that Alex should refuse the loop monitor. My son was pretty frustrated at this point because he felt they had put him through a lot.

The next day Alex was fine. There didn't seem to be anything more I could do for him, so I left to go help my daughter, who was moving into a college dorm room in another part of the state. Five days later Alex called and told us he had been given a clean bill of health at his follow-up visit with the family medicine doctor. I thought this was a little strange given that he had previously been told that they were going to look into the possibility of genetic testing. I think the family medicine doctor had not been told of this recommendation. Her records show that she told Alex that "there was nothing more they could do for him." Again, there was no mention of not running.

I continued to talk with Alex about his health. I thought he had a potassium problem, as his potassium had been low in the blood sample taken in the emergency room. Nothing had ever been done about this. I had talked to a nurse about the potassium level at the time and she said they were going to replace potassium for him. I also talked to the cardiologist who did the heart catheterization; he said the potassium was not too low and not to worry about it. However, that doctor did tell me that he was concerned that the electrocardiogram had showed that Alex's QT interval was a little long. This is a potentially dangerous heart rhythm disturbance that can lead to sudden death. I asked a few questions and realized that the QT interval is affected by the heart rate. Alex had a pretty low heart rate. I asked if this had been corrected for and they told me yes, it had been, but that the QT interval was still too long and this was worrisome. That was where we left it. I did not understand the significance of the long QT interval at the time.

Two and a half weeks after his outpatient visit with the family practitioner, my son went running alone in the evening and collapsed and died. Later we found out that a lifeguard had come by and given him CPR, but it was too late. Medics came and got his heart started, but it was too late. He was admitted to the hospital in a deep coma. Three days later his heart failed and he died.

My wife used those 3 days as a grace period. Our extended family and many friends came to be with us during this time. Alex's friends came from near and far and shared our grief. The impact of his death was widespread. People in our church community were mortified. His friends were mortified. Our whole family was mortified. The grief was like a pebble in a pond: it just radiated.

Reconstructing What Happened

After Alex died, I had a lot of questions. To provide some perspective on this, I have a PhD in pathology and am a board-certified toxicologist, but I did not know what to expect. I had been taught that medical records were "for physicians' eyes only." I was so fearful of trying to get my son's medical records that I went through a physician I knew from work. He requested them and we received a small stack of paper. We went to a lawyer, who said that there was no way that this was Alex's complete set of medical records, so my lawyer got a complete set for me.

I should note that it is not easy to look at your dead son's medical records. But I felt I did not have a choice. I had to know what had happened, not just for Alex's sake, but for his two siblings.

The first question I had was about the potassium level. From the beginning I thought that Alex's potassium level was a problem that was never recognized by the doctors. Two years before all this unfolded there had been a publication in the *Archives of Internal Medicine* by the National Council on Potassium in Clinical Practice. This article said that if a patient's potassium was below 4 mEq/L and that patient also had cardiac arrhythmias, then you must replace potassium and you must also consider replacing magnesium (Cohn, Kowey, Whelton, & Prisant, 2000).

That guideline was clearly missed by his doctors. Alex had a potassium of 3.4 mEq/L, not remarkably low, but he also had three arrhythmias, which were associated with increased risk of sudden cardiac death. He had frequent premature ventricular contractions (PVCs). Of the seven heartbeats recorded on the electrocardiogram after he collapsed the first time, two were PVCs. He also had a long QT interval. In fact, he scored 5.5 points on the widely published Schwartz diagnostic criteria for long QT syndrome. Anything over 4.0 on this scale is considered to indicate a high probability of having long QT syndrome (Khan, 2002). In Alex's case, I think this was quite probably acquired long QT syndrome caused by potassium depletion. Alex's doctors missed that diagnosis.

In fact, as amazing it seems to me, the first consultant said Alex's QT interval was normal. But there is no such thing as a normal QT interval. It cannot be judged normal until it is corrected for heart rate. Alex's corrected QT interval was quite elevated at 480 milliseconds. I actually took his electrocardiograms and measured them myself to confirm this. Given his collapse and other factors, he clearly should have been diagnosed with long QT syndrome.

When I saw Alex's complete medical records I was a little surprised to see that there was no record of his cardiac MRI scan. As you remember, the inconclusive cardiac MRI was the reason given for recommending a heart catheterization. I could not understand why the result of the MRI was not in the records. Then in April, 8 months after Alex had died, I got a call at work from a radiologist who said he could tell me some things about Alex's cardiac MRI that I might want to know. He told me that my son's cardiac MRI had been aborted. He said that, in fact, the hospital had recently introduced new software for their machine and the technical operators had not been trained on it.

The MRI had not been done properly. They never told us that while Alex was in the hospital. Alex could have had a cardiac MRI done in Dallas, where there was a doctor who regularly did them. The radiologist also said that Alex could have had the MRI repeated in the original hospital by people with the right skills. But this option was never given to us.

I also looked at the records from the hospital where my son had the electrophysiology test. Alex was small, about 155 pounds. He had been given nearly the maximum dose of the narcotic drug fentanyl and the sedative Versed, which is well known to cause amnesia. Then the record shows that they talked to us for 14 minutes about what he should and shouldn't do. I suppose they assumed that because I was there I would make sure that Alex knew not to run. They never told me that. I had no idea that the drugs he had been given would affect his memory, and I guarantee you that I did not mention not running after that because that was not what he wanted to hear.

The place for that instruction to my son would have been on the written instructions when we left the hospital. But the only thing that was written was, "Don't drive for 24 hours"—and he didn't. This was a huge mistake of situational awareness and communication. When a patient is discharged from a hospital, even on an outpatient basis, physicians have to be cognizant of what the patient is being told and what the patient understands.

The Standard of Care in Texas

We did not have a full autopsy conducted on my son, but they did a pathology study of his heart and brain. The brain was normal. His heart was sent to a pathologist in Dallas. The pathologist reported myocarditis—inflammation—in my son's heart and damage to the left ventricular septum, the wall separating the lower chambers of the heart. He was careful and did not say why the myocarditis occurred. There are infectious causes of myocarditis, which bloodwork showed was clearly not the case for Alex. But there are other causes of lesions identical to myocarditis, and one of them is potassium depletion. This fit with the low potassium evident in the electrolytes when Alex first went into the hospital.

One of the inaccuracies that I began to see flowing through Alex's medical records was the claim that he had been offered and refused a pacemaker, which might have prevented the arrhythmia that killed him. This was a false statement. Alex was offered a loop monitor, which does not regulate the heartbeat. The records from the second hospital and from the cardiology consultants show clearly that he was offered a loop monitor and not a pacemaker. I think the first cardiologist went back to his home hospital after my son died and told the other doctors that he had offered my son a pacemaker and they placed this in his records.

It was also in the records of the pathologist, which sent me through the ceiling because whether or not it is true, that does not belong in a pathologist's report. It was not his business what the patient was offered or not. I tried to get that man to take it out and he refused to do it. All I could get him to do was put documents from Alex's record in his files.

I corresponded with this pathologist over the years. He looked microscopically at what he called myocarditis. I wanted him to look at the lesion in the ventricular septum because I felt there was possibly an injury from the cardiac catheter. These injuries are pretty rare, but one thing I know from the medical records is that the cardiologist used a large catheter, and the fact that Alex had a large hematoma after the procedure also suggests that maybe it was not done very carefully. Of course, one can never prove these things, but at least you can see the age of the lesion if you take a microscopic section, and the pathologist refused to do this.

Eventually I went to the Texas Medical Board. They informed me that their cardiologist had deemed that my son's care met the standard of care in Texas. I thought that was ridiculous so I appealed, and I lost again. The next cardiologist said that my son's care exceeded the standard of care in Texas.

So my question is, "What is the standard of care in Texas?" I feel it's whatever the expert witness says it is. There is a huge disincentive for the medical board's reviewing physicians to find fault with another physician's care because they would have to say that one of their colleagues did not meet the standard of care, and that is confrontational and unpleasant. The point is that Alex's diagnosis of myocarditis never had to be made. Following the guidelines alone would have preserved my son's life.

Figure 7-1 outlines the events leading to Alex's death.

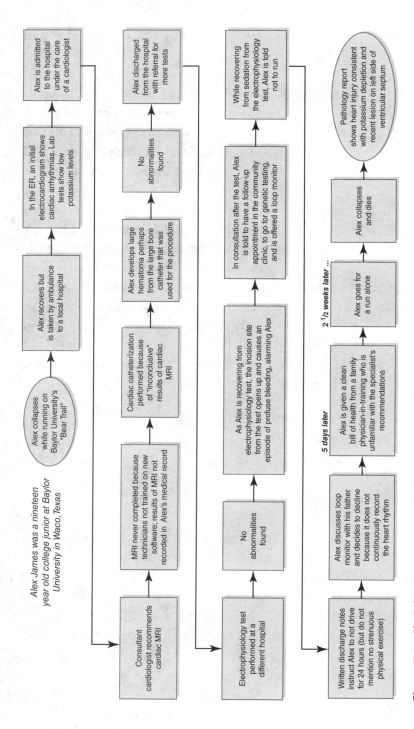

Figure 7-1. Alex's Story

Conclusion

A few years later I started thinking about what I should do about all this. I wrote a book called *A Sea of Broken Hearts* (James, 2007). It is for all the people who have died or been harmed in health care. My lessons for patients are simple. The first is to follow your intuition. If I had followed my intuition from the start maybe my son would be here now. My second piece of advice is to ask questions. Probably in hindsight I could have asked more hard questions the last time we were in the room with the doctors. I should not have assumed that they were going to hand my son off to a cardiologist for a hospital follow-up visit. I made that assumption and that was a mistake.

This is the final thing I would say to patients. There is danger out there and there is healing, and you do not want to get in the danger zone. I have seen a lot of effort to fix the system. Sadly, it does not seem to have had much impact. By my calculation, extrapolating from the most recently available studies, the incidence of death from medical harm in American hospitals is between 210,000 and 440,000 people every year (James, 2013). In my opinion the biggest flaw in all this is that there is not a concerted effort to engage patients and their advocates. The system needs to make the patient and his or her advocate full partners with full transparency. When we do that we will begin to make real progress, but I think we are a long way away from it yet.

Case Discussion

Alex James died from cardiac arrest several weeks after an earlier episode of syncope while running in the summer heat in central Texas. He almost certainly died of undiagnosed long QT syndrome, a disturbance of the heart's electrical activity that can cause sudden dangerous heart arrhythmias in response to exercise or other stresses (National Heart, Lung, and Blood Institute, 2011). Alex's father, John James, an experienced researcher, delved into the medical literature and his son's medical records to recreate the underlying causes of the trail of errors that he saw as leading to Alex's death.

Long QT syndrome is associated with electrolyte imbalances, particularly low potassium, which may be genetic, but which the literature confirms can also be brought on by strenuous exercise in hot, humid climates like that of central Texas. In unraveling the mystery of his son's death, John came to what he felt to be the inescapable conclusion that Alex had acquired long QT syndrome as a result of potassium depletion. He found it inexplicable that the diagnosis of long QT syndrome was not made in the face of considerable supporting evidence, and that even in the absence of a diagnosis his son was not given potassium supplementation in accord with current guidelines.

The issue that troubled John James most was his perception that the cardiologists in his son's case did not appear to be aware of current research and guidelines in their own field, a situation he believes is far from unique. He believes that maintenance of certification and other means of continuous learning are needed to correct this deficiency. Dr. James felt that his son was subjected to painful and invasive testing that had little chance of providing additional information, while the electrocardiogram and electrolyte test results that were the key to accurate diagnosis were not given serious consideration. This ties in with the observation by Newman-Toker, McDonald, and Melzer (2013) that the temptation to use available technology has led to a costly gap between what we "should do" and what we "actually do," but has done little to improve the rate of correct diagnosis. The result in Alex's case appears to have been that his doctors failed to adequately interpret available data and discharged Alex without precautions being taken against what turned out to be a fatal condition.

Questions

1. Discuss the requirements for maintenance of certification or maintenance of licensure in your field. What factors might prevent healthcare providers from following current

guidelines? What do you think is the best way to ensure that healthcare professionals' knowledge remains accurate and up-to-date?

2. Look up the Institute of Medicine's standards for guideline production. Do you think most existing guidelines meet these standards? How can a clinician assess the quality of existing guidelines? What should you do if you have doubts about the reliability of a guideline?

3. Research the incidence and causes of diagnostic error. How big a problem is this, and how can it be addressed? What factors do you think might have influenced Alex's diagnostic course?

4. Look up the elements that should be included in an informed consent discussion. How might adherence to the principles of transparency and informed consent have affected the choices of the James family?

5. Dr. James believes that one reason for his son's death while running was that Alex was given verbal discharge instructions while still under the influence of drugs with the potential to affect memory. As a consequence, he was unaware of the admonition not to run. What are the lessons for healthcare providers when providing instructions to patients and their families?

6. Which of the core competencies for health professions are most relevant for this case? Why?

References

Cohn, J. N., Kowey, P. R., Whelton, P. K., & Prisant, L. M. (2000). New guidelines for potassium replacement in clinical practice: A contemporary review by the National Council on Potassium in Clinical Practice. *Archives of Internal Medicine, 160*(16), 2429–2436.

James, J. T. (2013). A new, evidence-based estimate of patient harms associated with hospital care. *Journal of Patient Safety, 9*(3), 122–128.

James, J. T. (2007). *A sea of broken hearts: Patient rights in a dangerous, profit-driven health care system*. Bloomington: Authorhouse.

Khan, I. A. (2002). Long QT syndrome: Diagnosis and management. *American Heart Journal, 143*(1), 7–14.

National Heart, Lung, and Blood Institute, National Institutes of Health, U.S. Department of Health and Human Services. (2011). Long QT syndrome. Available at: https://www.nhlbi.nih.gov/health/health-topics/topics/qt/.

Newman-Toker, D. E., McDonald, K. M., & Melzer, D. O. (2013). How much diagnostic safety can we afford, and how should we decide? A health economics perspective. *BMJ Quality and Safety, 22*(Suppl 2), ii11–ii20.

Practice–Based Learning and Improvement

Healthcare professionals must demonstrate the ability to investigate and evaluate their care of patients, to appraise and assimilate scientific evidence, and to continuously improve patient care based on constant self-evaluation and lifelong learning. Specific competencies within the Practice-Based Learning and Improvement domain are to:

- Identify strengths, deficiencies, and limits in one's knowledge and expertise.
- Set learning and improvement goals.
- Identify and perform learning activities that address one's gaps in knowledge, skills, and/or attitudes.
- Systematically analyze practice using quality improvement methods, and implement changes with the goal of practice improvement.
- Incorporate feedback into daily practice.
- Locate, appraise, and assimilate evidence from scientific studies related to patients' health problems.
- Use information technology to optimize learning.

- Participate in the education of patients, families, students, trainees, peers, and other health professionals.
- Obtain and utilize information about individual patients, populations of patients, or communities from which patients are drawn to improve care.
- Continually identify, and implement new knowledge, guidelines, standards, technologies, products, or services that have been demonstrated to improve outcomes.

The three cases presented in Section 3 represent a wide array of patient harm in different clinical settings and patient populations. The cases are complex and include elements of other competencies as well. As you read the cases, think about the other competencies that are relevant. (Refer to the full list of competencies in the appendix.)

Case 8, "Improving Care for People with Intellectual Disability," is a case from Australia that is based on a teenage male with an intellectual disability and autism spectrum disorder. Andy lives in a group home, but escalating behavioral problems that the staff could not manage led to an emergency admission to the local hospital. This case highlights the potential implications of intellectual disability on communication, patient care, and patient safety. Andy's experience led to redesign of the care process, which is described in the case.

Case 9, "A Cascade of Small Events: Learning from an Unexpected Postsurgical Death," is the story of Nick Canfield from British Columbia, Canada, who underwent a surgical excision of a soft tissue sarcoma on his thigh. While recovering in the hospital, he developed delirium and became infected with *Clostridium difficile*. Nick died 8 days after he was admitted to the hospital.

Case 10, "Accidental Fall in a Hospital," tells the story of Colin Lake who was admitted to the eye ward of a hospital in Australia for an ulcer on his cornea. Colin's stay was lengthened and complicated by a fall outside the hospital that fractured his right wrist. After reviewing the event, the eye ward implemented changes to assess all patients for falls risk on admission and to classify every patient on intensive eye drop therapy as a high falls risk.

CASE 8

Improving Care for People with Intellectual Disability

The Story of Andy (Australia)

Deborah Debono, Jurgen Wille, David Skalicky, Julie Johnson,
Robert Leitner, and Bruce Chenoweth

Editors' Note

This case is based on Andy (not his real name) and his experience navigating the Australian healthcare system. Andy's case highlights the needs of people with intellectual disability (ID) and/or autism spectrum disorder (ASD) and the importance of dedicated processes and structures that accommodate their needs.

Intellectual disability is characterised by limitations in general intellectual functioning and difficulties in adaptive behavior, including social and practical skills, that are evident before age 18 (Wen, 1997). Challenging behavior is often associated with ID, and as a result caring for people with an ID can be complex and challenging (Matson & Shoemaker, 2009). There are immense social impacts for those with ID, their families and caregivers, and society as a whole. It is estimated that in developed countries 1–3 in 100 people have an ID (Katz & Lazcano-Ponce, 2008).

ID is often accompanied by psychopathological comorbidities, including mental illness. When compared with the general population, there is a higher prevalence of psychiatric and behavior disorders among people with an ID (Bradley, Summers, Wood, & Bryson, 2004). The autism and ASD subgroup is one of the largest diagnostic subgroups within the population of people with an ID (Matson & Shoemaker, 2009; Wilkins & Matson, 2009).[1]

---

[1] The Neurodevelopmental Work Group of the fifth edition of the *Diagnostic and Statistical Manual of Mental Disorders* (DSM-5) have proposed that the umbrella category, autism spectrum disorder, incorporate the previously separate diagnoses of autistic disorder, Asperger's disorder, childhood disintegrative disorder, and pervasive developmental disorder not otherwise specified.

ASD is characterized by difficulty with social interactions, communication (verbal and nonverbal), and repetitive behaviors (Autism Speaks, 2012). One of the key characteristics of ASD is the need for sameness (or lack of behavioral flexibility), particularly in specific situations (Green et al., 2006). Therefore, people with ASD need a highly structured and predictable social and care environment (Galli Carminati, Gerber, Baud, & Baud, 2007).

LEARNING OBJECTIVES

After completing this case study, you will be able to:

1. Discuss factors to consider in the management of a person with an intellectual disability.
2. Consider the effect of intellectual disability on communication, patient care, and patient safety.
3. Develop strategies for healthcare providers to accommodate for the needs of a person with an intellectual disability.

Andy's Story

Andy is a 17-year-old teenaged male with significant intellectual disability, autism, and a range of psychiatric and behavioral disorders. Andy was born in Sydney, Australia, and lived with his mother and younger sister for many years. Andy was formally assessed at the age of 4 and diagnosed as having an autistic disorder with moderate to severe intellectual disability. He has conductive hearing and sleeping problems likely due to obstructive sleep apnea. Andy's family is devoted to him, and like many families with a disabled child it has been a difficult road for them.

Andy is nonverbal, although basic communication is possible and visuals (e.g., hand signs and picture cards meaning "yes," "stop," and "more") are often used. Andy responds adversely to sensory overstimulation (e.g., auditory, physical, and visual modes). Sensory inputs such as simple sounds or lights or chaotic environments may cause distress, pain, or confusion or simply cause him to be overwhelmed. Some inputs may be interesting to him, but when interrupted without warning, these inputs will cause distress. When overwhelmed, Andy will decompensate. He will employ self-soothing behaviors such as whole-body movements, rocking, and repetitive slapping on his thigh. Andy's performs best when he is in a well-defined routine with familiar surroundings and around people he knows and trusts.

Andy started at a school for children with intellectual and physical disabilities when he was 6 years old. Over time, his behavior became more and more violent, antagonistic, and unmanageable, with increasing negative impact on his sister. The decision was made to move Andy into respite care for a few days a week. Later he was moved to a weekly boarding school coupled intermittently with temporary care. Finally, when Andy was 15 years old, he was moved to permanent residential care in a group home.

Over the years, Andy's behavior has fluctuated with extremely challenging, aggressive, violent bouts; unusual behaviors, including crawling and other bizarre postures; laughing inappropriately and in response to some internal stimuli; together with preoccupation with various obsessions and compulsions and self-injurious behavior. Examples of Andy's challenging behaviors include climbing on kitchen cupboards, window sills, and the car. A multidisciplinary approach was used to manage Andy, incorporating the use of diet and exercises to decrease his hypersensitivity to stimuli. Andy has been treated by an array of practitioners, including a pediatric psychiatrist, a psychologist, a general practitioner, a sleep physician, a social worker, and an occupational therapist. The practitioners from the specialist ID health team provide a comprehensive and coordinated range of community-based services that have minimized the need for acute hospital presentations. A relationship has been carefully built among Andy's mother; mental health services; Ageing, Disability, and Home Care (ADHC) services; and the disability specialist services. Andy has been treated with a regimen of medications, including, but not limited to, haloperidol (Serenace), mirtazapine (Avanza), amisulpride (Solian), dexamphetamine, methyl phenidate (Ritalin), risperidone (Risperdal), clonidine (Catapress), sodium valproate (Epilim), and

---

Box 8-1 Profile of Mercy Hospital

Mercy Hospital is a large, quaternary metropolitan teaching hospital renowned for its ability to treat complex and difficult conditions. It receives emergency referrals from throughout the state and also services the local population. Mercy Hospital has a very hospital-centric administrative approach tailored toward critical care and specialized, high-technology services. It provides little in the way of outreach and offers limited networks with community support services for people with ID.

---

olanzapine (Zyprexa). The medications have had mixed effects with many side effects ranging from acting out, involuntary movements to extreme appetite and weight gain.

All aspects of Andy's care are highly regulated: for example, he only takes his medication with orange juice and for lunch he eats vegemite sandwiches cut in half with no crusts. The group home provides good structure and consistency, however, it is in a new urban area which is at a distance from Andy's home, local school, and mental health and disability health services where he was well known. Although the aim was to identify and engage with new local providers, Andy continued to receive support from his previous specialist ID health team who knew him well and continued to be available for formal consultations and informal telephone contact.

Andy's history incorporates severe escalations in violent and self-injurious behavior, resulting in presentations to the emergency department (ED) at two different hospitals: Lakeview Hospital (see **Box 8-1**) and Mercy Hospital (see **Box 8-2**). The two hospitals are teaching hospitals affiliated with state universities and are well regarded for the healthcare services they provide.

Box 8-2 Profile of Lakeview Hospital

Lakeview Hospital began as a small hospital and has developed over the years to become one of the largest hospitals in the state, providing an array of specialist healthcare services. Lakeview is a disability community service-based hospital. It has a strong relationship with a proactive specialist ID health team, local community support services, and local general practitioner services that are familiar with the particular needs of people with ID. When hospitalization is necessary, Lakeview Hospital seeks support from the specialist ID health team and aims to provide patient-centered care for a person with an ID. To this end, it continues to develop local capacity and to implement processes and protocols that cater for the unique needs of a person with an ID.

Andy's presentations to the ED have been precipitated by a variety of reasons, including restlessness due to withdrawal from haloperidol (a dopamine antagonist used in the treatment of autism). The sudden withdrawal of haloperidol can cause excitation of suppressed motor pathways, leading to extreme agitation and motor restlessness. This resulted in extremely challenging behavior, including screaming, an inability to sit still, and hitting himself violently. Andy's autism makes presentation to the ED particularly difficult because he has a heightened perception of his environment and sensory inputs, including visual, auditory, olfactory, and tactile. He is unable to process the complex simultaneous sensory input of the ED environment, which causes him to become panicky and anxious in those settings. The sensory load of the ED and extended wait time in an unfamiliar environment escalates challenging behavior and causes Andy to become very distressed, increasing the chance that he will lash out.

Andy's Hospitalizations

Andy's complex needs have led to multiple hospital presentations. Two of these presentations to two different hospitals are described below.

Scenario 1: Mercy Hospital

For the first time in his new group home, Andy had been displaying a steady increase in self-injurious behaviors and property damage. The caregivers at the group home were neither able to manage the behavior nor administer medication as prescribed. It was early Friday of a holiday weekend. The caregivers tried calling Andy's general practitioner (GP), whom he sees regularly; however, she was away that weekend. They felt that their only option was to send him to the hospital. They called an ambulance and informed his mother. The ambulance team struggled to restrain Andy, and accompanied by one of the group home caregivers they took him to the nearest ED at Mercy Hospital.

Andy was extremely agitated and very distressed in the ED. The ED was busy and noisy, with computer screens, bright halogen lights above, and large numbers of staff and patients moving about. Andy's wailing and self-injurious and aggressive behavior escalated; he pushed over a sharps cart, bit his own hand, and slapped the arm of staff when they tried to put on a blood pressure cuff. Two hospital security staff were called to help restrain Andy. As his behavior escalated further, Andy spat his oral Zyprexa at them and started throwing items from the bedside. A junior registrar and nurse arrived, and the four staff restrained him while a dose of intramuscular midazolam was given. While still restrained in bed, droperidol and ketamine were prescribed in incremental doses. Andy then suddenly became quite sleepy and flaccid, and stopped breathing. The cardiac arrest team was called, and Andy was intubated, stabilized and transferred to the intensive care unit (ICU).

Andy remained intubated overnight in the ICU, and his mother stayed with him in the hospital. When he was extubated the following day, he awoke acutely distressed and agitated. His behavior started to escalate again, and Andy was quickly transferred to the psychiatric ward where he was placed in a locked seclusion room with his mother and a worker. During his hospitalization, Andy continued to be agitated, refused to take his medication, and would not eat his meals. At one point, while in the locked room, Andy hit his mother dislodging her tooth. As the holiday weekend came to an end, Andy's specialist ID health team was notified with a request to transfer Andy by ambulance to Lakeview Hospital. On the strong advice of the team, he was discharged back to the group home. **Figure 8-1** provides an overview of Andy's 4-day hospitalization.

According to a social worker involved with the case, "When Andy was discharged he was very unsettled, so from what we know he was highly traumatized."

Scenario 2: Lakeview Hospital

As part of the discharge planning from Mercy hospital, Andy's mother, the group home staff, and the local disability support staff

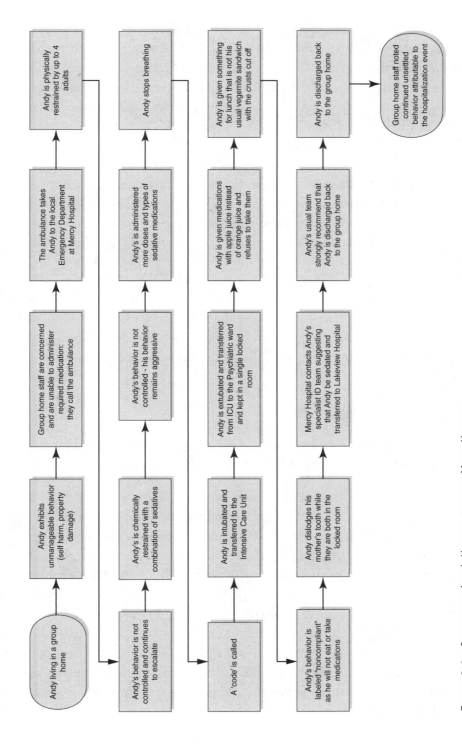

FIGURE 8-1. OVERVIEW OF ANDY'S HOSPITALIZATION AT MERCY HOSPITAL

requested help from the specialist ID health team (located in the area where Andy previously lived). The team had an established, supportive relationship with Lakeview Hospital and a good understanding of Andy's medical and psychosocial needs. They met to discuss Andy's case and how to prevent a similar situation from happening in the future. Transitions between care settings—from group home to ED, from ED to inpatient ward, and from inpatient ward back to group home—were particularly vulnerable times for Andy's care. They agreed that because of Andy's altered perception of his environment, he would react strongly to sensory inputs, such as visual, auditory, olfactory, and tactile inputs. His responses are augmented by his ID, which made him panicky and anxious in unfamiliar settings, causing him to lash out. Andy's distress and anxiety during the ED presentation at Mercy Hospital were amplified by his care deviating from his routine and an inability to communicate verbally. The lights and sounds of the ED contributed to the escalation of his behavior, which was then further exacerbated by the physical restraints. As his social worker notes:

Some of the behaviors were actually a result of the admission itself, not the reason for it. People with autism are aligned on rigid rules that they apply universally, and their intuitive capacity is really impaired. It is important to consider the information provided by their nonverbal cues. With Andy there was no hint of physical pain, and no obvious evidence of psychotic behavior.

The team were motivated to consider ways to improve the process to accommodate Andy's needs. Their established relationship with Lakeview Hospital and their ability to support change and develop capacity empowered the team to suggest improvements to better handle ED presentation and hospitalization of people with an ID. One process change proposed was to subvert the usual triage process with direct admission. Ideally an alert would be included on Andy's medical record to signal to the ED staff about Andy's particular needs. This alert would trigger the option of an alternative triage process for Andy; for example, he would be taken directly to a quiet room to minimize the impact of the ER sensory load. Implementing this trigger system poses logistical challenges requiring process and technical changes (e.g., creating a new field in the electronic medical record [EMR]) and would take time to roll out. Furthermore, success would depend on the ability of the clinicians to identify whether the person presenting at the ED has an ID, which may be difficult, particularly in cases of mild ID.

Andy's hospitalization required engaging his caregivers in the discharge plans, including case conferences with hospital staff, group home staff, family/caregivers, and community disability services to support communication and care management during the hospitalization and discharge process.

Several weeks later, Andy's behavior was unmanageable and progressively escalated. He was agitated, screaming, hitting himself, and could not sit still. It was evident from his behavior that Andy would not be able to sit in the ED waiting room. Andy's mother took him to the specialist ID health team connected with Lakeview Hospital. Because there is an established relationship between the specialist ID health team and Lakeview Hospital, his psychiatrist escorted Andy to the ED and the normal triage process was subverted. In its place, an alternative triage process fast tracked Andy through the ED waiting room, and he was taken to a quiet room. Andy remained extremely agitated, but, in contrast to his previous ED experience at Mercy Hospital, this time he did not need to be physically restrained. Andy was admitted to the hospital and was accommodated in a quiet room at the end of the medical ward. The single patient room was located at the end of a corridor, thus reducing the traffic flow around the room. The lights in the room could be dimmed and the noises and stimulation from the equipment, lights, and hustle and bustle of the rest of the hospital could be minimized. The location of the single room meant that it was possible to employ unobtrusive attendance of security personnel, thus reducing the likelihood of agitation and confrontation. Andy's mother was able to stay and offer comfort and help interpret Andy's needs and gestures.

As Andy's condition improved, it was recognized that a time buffer was needed to ensure that the local networks that supported Andy were prepared for his discharge. To support Andy's discharge, the following processes were implemented: the local disability services office was informed of the planned date of discharge; Andy's discharge medications and paperwork were ready and on the ward prior to the discharge date; and strategies were implemented to support the group home and other local services involved in Andy's care. On the day of discharge, the manager drove Andy to the group home. Organizing Andy's transport allowed time to arrange the discharge and avoided delays that may have caused him further agitation. Andy was discharged to the group home and settled back into his routine quickly without the traumatization exhibited following the initial hospitalization. These processes were enabled by the strong relationships that the specialist ID health team had developed with the local community-based support networks. **Figure 8-2** outlines the process of care at Lakeview Hospital.

Conclusion

Andy's need for routine underscored the need to be discharged to an established venue. Failure to do so increased Andy's anxiety and consequent behavioral escalation. This was enabled by the connections among the hospital, the specialist ID health team, and the community support services. Andy's experience highlights the problems that may arise when people with complex and interwoven behavioral issues interface with a nonintegrated healthcare system. The importance of co-production of healthcare plans with the patients, caregivers, and community-based providers is essential. Patients with ID and ASD have specific requirements, some of which lend themselves to the introduction of policies and guidelines that shape service delivery. For example, the introduction of policies and structures that allow for the screening and identification of clients with ID and ASD and that enable them to bypass the usual ED triage process, shorten wait time, and provision of a room or area with reduced sensory load would benefit the majority of clients with ID and ASD. However, it is also imperative that clinicians understand that there are individually specific ID- and ASD-related needs that are pivotal to the delivery

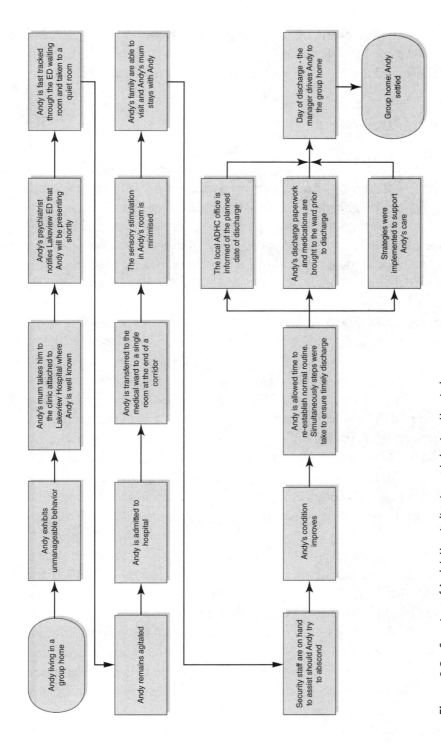

Figure 8-2. Overview of Andy's Hospitalization at Lakeview Hospital

of care (e.g., the client's preference for orange juice to take medication). The use of interpreter services for clients from non-English speaking backgrounds is widely implemented in health care.

Case Discussion

Worldwide, the prevalence of ASD has been increasing during the last few decades, with the variation in the prevalence reflecting a broadening of the diagnostic criteria, increased awareness in the general community, and diagnostic switching from a developmental disorder to ASD. The median of the worldwide prevalence estimate for the narrower diagnosis of autistic disorder is 17 in every 10,000 people, and the broader diagnosis of ASD is 62 in every 10,000 people, with a substantial variability across studies (Williams et al., 2008; Elsabbagh et al., 2012). The needs for people with both ID and ASD are different from those with either ID or ASD (Gilchrist et al., 2001; Galli Carminati et al., 2007; Boucher, Bigham, Mayes, & Muskett, 2008).

Sound principles must be in place when caring for people with ASD and/or ID. Activities must be highly regulated, and the person's particular preferences for the way things are done must be attended to. For example, according to a social worker familiar with Andy's first hospital admission, "Andy's mother is the interpreter of a very particular language, and the gate keeper of essential information relevant to the success of Andy's care. However, the importance of her basic instructions was not appreciated and they were not adhered to."

Best practice includes regular consultation with caregivers in acute care settings so that basic needs can be met. This is intensified for people with ASD. For example, "What do I look for if I want to know if Andy is in pain?" and "What does he like to do that keeps him engaged while in the hospital?" The important thing is to ask the questions and to consult the caregiver. Even with acknowledgment of the role of the caregiver in policy directives, in practice the caregiver perspective and input is often not recognized or explicitly solicited. Andy's mother was aware of his routines, such as the need for a vegemite sandwich with no crust for lunch and that he would only take medications with orange juice. Although this seems like a minor issue, for someone with ASD it can be vital information. In the initial scenario, the hospital providers were not aware of the importance of this issue for Andy's medication adherence. **Table 8-1** summarizes some best practice characteristics for providing care to people with ID (United Nations, 2006).

Healthcare systems are complex, with unpredictability and uncertainty contributing to the difficulty of delivering patient-centered care in even straightforward cases. ID and ASD add another layer of complexity that requires a shift in the current mental models regarding the delivery of care to those with ID. Andy's experience emphasizes

Table 8-1 Best Practice Characteristics in ID Care

Best Practice	Comments
Accessible	• Facilities readily usable by a person with a disability. • Services reasonably and equitably provided irrespective of the disability.
Avoidable hospitalizations	• Prevention of unnecessary hospital admission by providing timely and efficient support in the community.
Caregiver aware	• Awareness, recognition, support, and appreciation of the many caregivers who provide unpaid care and support to the family.
Choice in treatments	• Maximized involvement of people with a disability and their caregivers in their health care.
Community support	• Service provided to people with a disability in their local community.
Disability action plan	• An organization's written commitment to achieving and implementing plans to improve access to services and facilities for people with a disability.
Disability awareness	• Understanding of issues surrounding disability with a focus on the individual, not the disability. • Understanding of appropriate and effective methods of communication with people with disabilities.
Discharge planning	• Comprehensive, coordinated approach to discharge from the hospital and follow-up with patients in a process that involves the patient, caregiver/family, and community-support services.

(continued)

Table 8-1 Best Practice Characteristics in ID Care *(continued)*

Best Practice	Comments
Flexible services	• Services that adapt their processes and protocols to be responsive to the holistic needs of the individual.
Health management plan	• Document that specifies the person's healthcare needs, management, and treatment plans.
Holistic approach	• Comprehensive approach to service delivery and treatment with coordination of the patient's overall care and well-being as the priority.
Hospitalization guidelines	• Good practice guidelines for managing the patient with intellectual disability in emergency departments.
Human rights	• Respect for the rights and dignity of persons with disabilities.
Inclusion in mainstream	• The inclusion of people with disabilities in programs, activities, and facilities with their nondisabled peers.
Integrated services	• Coordinated hospital and community-based services that link intake, assessment, crisis intervention, and acute, extended and ongoing treatment using a case management approach to ensure continuity of care.
Interagency networks	• Effective interagency partnerships to meet the variety of educational, social, and health needs of people with disabilities and their caregivers.
Multidisciplinary teams	• Specialist multidisciplinary intellectual disability health team providing comprehensive specialist assessment and ongoing medical management of patients with chronic and complex health needs.
Person-centered care	• The focus is on the individual at the center of the service delivery process. • Working with person with intellectual disability and caregiver/support person as partners in care.
Prevention	• Early identification and intervention to minimize and prevent further disabilities.
Primary care involvement	• The general practitioner as the primary clinician who shares care with the specialist hospital and community-based services.

United Nations. (2006). "Convention on the Rights of Persons with Disabilities." Retrieved 2nd April, 2013, from http://www.un.org/disabilities/convention/conventionfull.shtml

the potential problems associated with imposing generic hospitalization processes, responses, and protocols on people with ID or ASD. This case study also offers examples of process changes that have improved the hospitalization experiences for this population group. In highlighting potential issues associated with hospital presentation for this population, we encourage the development of targeted systems that address the needs of this particularly vulnerable population group.

Questions

1. What were the system failures in Andy's care process?

2. How did the hospitals differ in their demonstrated understanding of the specific health needs of the patient in light of his disability?

3. What was the significance of the partnerships and networks among the family, group home, specialist ID health team, and Lakeview Hospital for Andy's hospitalization experiences?

4. What were the triage processes and protocols in both EDs that enabled or acted as barriers to Andy receiving effective care?

5. Are there other process improvements that you would consider to improve Andy's hospitalization experience?

6. How do the current handover requirements of information about patients meet the information handover needs for people with an intellectual disability?

7. How does the use of a disability action plan and discharge plan influence the hospital care of a person with ID or ASD?

8. What can we learn from this case about the importance of designing strategies and/or tools to engage patients, caregivers, and their families?

9. Which of the core competencies for health professions are most relevant for this case? Why?

References

American Psychiatric Association. (2013). *Diagnostic and statistical manual of mental disorders, Fifth edition (DSM-5)*. Washington, DC: Author.

Autism Speaks. (2012). What is autism? What is autism spectrum disorder?" Available at: http://www.autismspeaks.org/what-autism.

Boucher, J., Bigham, S., Mayes, A., & Muskett, T. (2008). Recognition and language in low functioning autism. *Journal of Autism and Developmental Disorders, 38*(7), 1259–1269.

Bradley, E., Summers, J., Wood, H. L., & Bryson, S. E. (2004). Comparing rates of psychiatric and behavior disorders in adolescents and young adults with severe intellectual disability with and without autism. *Journal of Autism and Intellectual Disorders, 34*(2), 151–161.

Elsabbagh, M., Divan, G., Koh, Y. J., Kim, Y. S., Kauchali, S., Marcin, C., . . . Fombonne, E. (2012). Global prevalence of autism and other pervasive developmental disorders. *Autism Research, 5*(3), 160–179.

Galli Carminati, G., Gerber, F., Baud, M. A., & Baud, O. (2007). Evaluating the effects of a structured program for adults with autism spectrum disorders and intellectual disabilities. *Research in Autism Spectrum Disorders, 1*(3), 256–265.

Gilchrist, A., Green, J., Cox, A., Burton, D., Rutter, M., & Le Couteur, A. (2001). Development and current functioning in adolescents with Asperger syndrome: A comparative study. *Journal of Child Psychology and Psychiatry, 42*(2), 227–240.

Green, V., Sigafoos, J., Pituch, K. A., Itchon, J., O'Reilly, M., & Lancioni, G. E. (2006). Assessing behavioral flexibility in individuals with developmental disabilities. *Focus on Autism and Other Developmental Disabilities, 21*(4), 230–236.

Katz, G., & Lazcano-Ponce, E. (2008). Intellectual disability: Definition, etiological factors, classification, diagnosis, treatment and prognosis. *Salud Pública de México, 50*(2), 132–141.

Matson, J. L., & Shoemaker, M. (2009). Intellectual disability and its relationship to autism spectrum disorders. *Research in Developmental Disabilities, 30*(6), 1107–1114.

United Nations. (2006). Convention on the Rights of Persons with Disabilities. Available at: http://www.un.org/disabilities/convention/conventionfull.shtml.

Wen, X. (1997). The definition and prevalence of intellectual disability in Australia. Australian Institute of Health and Welfare, Canberra. AIHW Catalogue no. DIS 2.

Wilkins, J., & Matson, J. (2009). A comparison of social skills profiles in intellectually disabled adults with and without ASD. *Behaviour Modification, 33*, 143–155.

Williams, K., MacDermott, S., Ridley, G., Glasson, E. J., & Wray, J. A. (2008). The prevalence of autism in Australia. Can it be established from existing data?" *Journal of Paediatrics and Child Health, 44*(9), 504–510.

A Cascade of Small Events: Learning from an Unexpected Postsurgical Death

The Story of Nick Francis (Canada)

Carolyn Canfield

Editors' Note

Carolyn Canfield is a former researcher and community organizer who resides in the Gulf Islands of British Columbia, Canada. Carolyn and her husband Nick Francis, a retired Royal Canadian Air Force chief flying instructor, worked for 20 years as active volunteers in their close-knit island community. The couple's lives changed abruptly when Nick, at the age of 79, discovered a lump on the back of his thigh. Doctors identified it as soft tissue sarcoma, a serious and relatively rare cancer that comprises less than 1% of all adult cancers. Standard treatment for soft tissue sarcoma in the extremities is surgical removal, often preceded and/or followed by radiation, chemotherapy, or a combination of the two (Burningham, Hashibe, Spector, & Schiffman, 2012). Nick underwent radiation followed by surgical excision of the tumor in a nearby hospital. While recovering in the hospital, he developed delirium and a Clostridium difficile infection. Hospital staff were shocked when he died on his eighth night after admission. Carolyn Canfield describes the events of Nick's hospitalization and her quest to improve health care by focusing on restoring relationships and trust between patients and providers.

LEARNING OBJECTIVES

After completing this case study, you will be able to:

1. Outline the system issues that were revealed in Nick's case.
2. Discuss the problem of fragmentation in health care and ways that it can be minimized.
3. Create a strategy to elicit patient input in achieving high-quality health care.
4. Discuss ways to handle recognition of avoidable patient harm and disclosure of adverse events in hospitals.

The Perfect Patient

In the spring of 2008 my husband Nick had a biopsy that revealed a malignancy in a lump on the back of his thigh. Nick met with a surgeon, and they agreed that surgery was the best option for recovery. He had preoperative radiation, and we prepared for the surgery confident that we had a great team of healthcare practitioners. We had enormous respect for the way we had been treated. The surgery was scheduled to last 3 hours but in fact took 7 hours. The surgeon said it took a little longer than expected, but that things went great.

I saw Nick when he came out of recovery. He was groggy, but said he was happy that "the cutting part" was over. The next day the surgeon came in and asked him to move his foot around for mobility and for strength. Everything looked great. The surgeon was delighted that even with removing a hamburger-sized tumor from the back of his thigh and rearranging some muscles the prospects looked good that Nick would walk. Nick had a sip of broth and learned how to use an incentive spirometer to clear his lungs. It was a really good day.

The next morning I came back to the hospital early, around 7:00 a.m. My husband was wild-eyed and greeted me with, "Thank God you're here." He then explained to me that diarrhea and nausea had started in the middle of the night and he had not been able to get any rest. He was also distressed by vivid imagery every time he closed his eyes: when his eyes were open he was the person I knew and loved, but when he tried to sleep delirium brought on images that kept him awake. He was frightened and uncomfortable and embarrassed to need assistance to get on and off the bedpan so often. The leg surgery meant staying immobilized in bed. The occupational therapist had spoken hopefully about leg dangling, learning to walk, and plans for release in a week. Now it seemed this was going to be delayed.

It took 3 days of suffering diarrhea and nausea, then fever, before Nick's fecal sample was sent to the lab. It came back quickly with a diagnosis of *Clostridium difficile*, an intestinal infection that is highly transmissible in hospitals. Immediately, I was taught contact precautions of gowning, gloving, and masking. Nick's IV was placed on a pole, and we rolled his bed down to the end of the hall, where he was put into an isolation room in the burn unit.

Nick was treated for 4 days for *C. difficile* and after about 2 and a half days his symptoms were beginning to show signs of improvement. Meanwhile, he had a consult for blood in the urine and a few other things. I trusted the practitioners. I felt that everybody cared. However, I was concerned about the fact that his overall breathing was declining rather than improving and that he was getting weaker. He was still not sleeping, and he was not being given any food.

The eighth day after surgery, Nick died in the middle of the night. At the time he died he had not eaten for 8 days. He had slept perhaps 5 good solid hours in the last 6 days of his life. Nevertheless, his was not an expected death. The staffers caring for him were devastated.

Nick and I were 20 years apart in age and had taken every advantage of 35 fabulous years together. Through all those 35 years, because of our age difference, we had talked about the possibility of my outliving him. So when I learned that he had died, I was not as shocked as I might have been, but the timing was not what we had expected. In that moment I felt the axis of the earth shift ever so slightly, and I knew nothing in my life was going to be the same after that.

I arrived at the hospital at 6:00 a.m., just before the shift change. The night nurse whom I had known from the previous night shift was waiting for me outdoors, guessing correctly where I might try to enter so early in the day. She gave me a huge embrace and cried, whispering to me that Nick did not suffer. Then we went upstairs where I was allowed to stay with Nick's corpse as long as I wanted. Within a few minutes the day shift came on. By the time they walked into the reception area, the two nurses were completely overwhelmed with sobs. I embraced them and patted them on the back and assured them that Nick had had a wonderful life and had achieved far more than he ever thought he might. He had no dreams unsatisfied. After I had held both nurses for a while, I sort of felt a soap box rising under my feet, and I talked to the assembled nursing staff about how it was okay for me because I understood death was a part of life. I told them how grateful we both had been for the brilliant care we had had and that Nick had been so appreciative for their taking such good care of him and being so concerned for his well-being. I spent another 4 hours or so with Nick's body, and that was an important thing for me. I always thought something like that would be disturbing, but it was good to be with the body that I knew so well, and to learn so plainly that the person I loved had already left.

The gastroenterologist came to offer his condolences while I was still in the room with Nick. I had expressed some concern earlier about substandard cleaning and about erroneous instructions I had been given. For example, I had been told to wear a mask as part of contact precautions, but I learned on the Internet that *C. difficile* precautions don't consider transmission by air. The specialist said my observations were legitimate and that I shouldn't think that because I was not a medical person that what I said was irrelevant. The other thing I told him was that I really wanted to make a difference. I wanted to salvage something good out of this unexpected death that might help another patient, and Nick would want that, too.

The physician told me he would help me if I wanted to pursue this. I was very grateful for that encouragement. Within a week I returned to the hospital's acute care ward where Nick had first been after surgery. One of the nurses who had cared for him in his first few days recognized me. She expressed her condolences and said this was quite tragic. I asked her how she had found out that Nick had died. She said she found out about his death in the nurses' coffee room. I thought, "Man, this is terrible." These nurses were shocked about what had happened to a patient who was in their care, but they had no way of knowing about it except through hospital gossip.

Analyzing the Causes

A few weeks later I requested Nick's chart. I wanted to know what had happened and how to interpret the autopsy report I knew was coming. But I had no medical knowledge, so I talked to Nick's and my former family physician, who had retired but was still living in our community. We also had a couple of nurse friends who were anxious to learn how their friend Nick had died and were willing to help me decipher the chart. So I met with each of them. I was absolutely taken aback when one of the nurses said the signs were all there that Nick was getting ready to crash. She said, "At this point in my hospital, Nick would have been in the intensive care unit."

The more I learned about what Nick's medical experience actually had been, the more I realized that these preventable "complications" in care happen every day. The fact that he died might have been an unusually dramatic outcome, but postoperative delirium was predictable for a 79-year-old male with the typical comorbidities that he had. We were never aware that postoperative delirium could be lethal. I thought about his deteriorating respiration, his immobility in bed, his starvation, his hallucinations that prevented sleep. I'm no medical person, but it seemed to me that mobility, breathing, eating, and sleeping are pretty fundamental to health and recovery. These factors were not consistently tracked in my husband's chart.

I felt that the care plan for Nick was fragmented, narrowly matching symptoms to specialties, yet missing the continuous arc of experience of the patient. Patient safety researchers often use James Reason's "Swiss cheese model" to refer to the causes of medical harm, arguing that active and latent causes must line up, like holes in slices of Swiss cheese, to create the circumstances for an unexpected outcome. But it seemed to me that in Nick's case each slice was way more hole than cheese and that the opportunity for disaster was far greater than it should have been.

One thing that Nick often said to me was that catastrophes in aviation happen as a cascade of small events. The danger is that once the cascade starts, there is nothing you can do to halt it. You can't think quickly enough to begin to roll it back. I think that is precisely what happened with Nick. He experienced a number of dangerous conditions that were all associated with each other, compounded each other, and eventually became a cascade that was very difficult to stop. By the time the danger to the patient was recognized, there wasn't enough time to figure out exactly what was happening and what should be done to rescue Nick.

The autopsy came back and to my surprise he had bled to death. He had experienced a massive GI (gastrointestinal) hemorrhage. There were microlesions in his duodenum that had filled his small intestine and colon with freshly clotted blood. His heart had stopped due to inadequate blood supply.

Pushing Every Step of the Way

Astonished at hearing nothing more from the system, I conducted my own version of a root cause analysis. I wanted to help the system learn while I healed, so I needed to build partnerships with the practitioners. But I had to push every step of the way.

I decided that I needed to interview his caregivers. I did this not so much to find out why Nick died as to find out more about why the system did not work well. It was certainly not working well for these people who were so affected by Nick's death but were given so little information. And if a patient dies unexpectedly and there are care quality questions coming out of the chart, I thought I needed to do something to fix this gap.

I made appointments with each of his clinicians. I asked them really general questions like, "What is wrong in healthcare?" "What's wrong in the system you work in?" "Who makes the decisions?" "What makes them make a decision on that?" and "How can I influence their decision making?" I was struck by their organizational naiveté. It seemed to me that healthcare workers were not very strategically astute, in the sense of understanding how power is used and distributed in their system.

A problem arose when I interviewed the surgeon. I asked him about Nick's discharge summary, which was only a paragraph long. The first few sentences of the summary explained the surgery and did so accurately and concisely. But the second half, about the postoperative experience, was full of errors, omissions, and misleading assessments of Nick's care. The stated cause of death was wrong, with no mention of the GI bleed. It said Nick died of cardiorespiratory failure and indicated that I had declined an autopsy. In fact I had immediately signed the release for the autopsy that was then ordered and performed.

The surgeon was also the head of quality improvement for surgery. Gently, without trying to be aggressive, I asked him if he could correct the discharge information, because I wanted Nick's chart to be correct in case it should ever be screened for a retrospective study or research. I wanted Nick's way of dying to have a chance of becoming accurate "data" for learning. The surgeon told me, "I do not take directions from family members." I was astounded. I asked him if Nick's case had been reviewed by anyone but him. He said, "No."

Clearly, in the surgeon's eyes, Nick's death did not result from surgical error and therefore did not concern him or contain lessons for him or his colleagues. This surgeon was Nick's "most responsible physician," but he had not taken real stewardship of Nick's postoperative experience. The silos of specialties got in the way of comprehensive care and no one was really responsible for the patient.

Two years later, I presented Nick's case as part of a conference on medical ethics and disclosure of unanticipated medical outcomes. The hospital's chief executive officer was in the audience. Some people in the room were resistant to my narrative and analysis, but others saw value in it and were very welcoming. I gave my 20-minute talk and I could feel the tension in the room. The CEO attempted to apologize and I kind of cut him off. I told him there had never been a review of this case and to my best understanding an effective apology can only take place if you know what you are apologizing for. He quickly agreed. He invited me back a few weeks later and offered both a written and an oral apology.

At that point, I very much understood that this whole thing was a bit of a dance. It was a ritual that was necessary as much for the health authority as it was for me. I had accounted for my experience, and now the health authority had to account for its experience. I think we succeeded in reaching an understanding, but only partially. The understanding within the health authority about Nick's death is still woefully incomplete. The apology was also, therefore, quite incomplete. The practitioners who were involved have never met to review the case and so still have limited appreciation of what Nick's journey was to death and what their role may have been in it. Learning from this tragedy never occurred.

Conclusion

Since Nick's death, I have committed myself to full-time patient advocacy. I think that the challenges in healthcare quality have everything to do with creating an opportunity for patients and practitioners to reconnect. Change happens collaboratively. It happens with shared understanding. I think that at its core, health care is all about relationships and trust. Nick and I had complete optimistic faith in the quality of the health care that was ahead of us. Betrayal of that trust has been my largest wound. This is what I struggle to recover from. We trusted and respected, and it was not returned.

The core of the problem is that healthcare providers are not able to see the patient as a whole. I think that if today we gathered Nick's 8 or 10 main healthcare providers into a room—the lead nurses, the specialists, and the surgeon—they would have a difficult time recalling the case. They might remember me and Nick, but they wouldn't be able to reconstruct the care experience because it was so fragmented. I saw the case, I reviewed the case, but nobody else saw it as a continuous joined-up patient experience of care. To them, there was a single discrete event: an unexpected, unfortunate death in the hospital. They didn't see anything to review.

We talk of wanting patient-centered care and of good patient outcomes as a measure of success. But only the patient can tell you if the outcome is good. Only the patient can tell you what matters and if the expectation was met. For change in health care to succeed, we need to plug in patient voices from boardroom to bedside; we need to empower patients in the care plan itself. If health care is about patients, then patients have to be involved in the design and the delivery and the governance of health care (Canfield, 2013). Connecting the patient to the healthcare treatment and delivery experience is huge for me. I don't have all the answers, but I know that, collectively, the patients have the answers. Patients are the experts in the patient experience.

Case Discussion

Carolyn Canfield raises several issues in her discussion of her husband's case. The first is what she sees as the extreme fragmentation of the healthcare system, preventing healthcare providers from seeing their patients as complete persons and from understanding their care as a whole. One consequence she sees is that the inability to follow a patient's case in its entirety can prevent healthcare providers from seeing the consequences of their contribution to care, and therefore prevent them from recognizing and preventing the causes of harm. As an example of this, she cites the lack of systematic charting of variables that she considers to have been significant contributors to her husband's decline: malnutrition, lack of sleep, lack of mobility, and delirium.

Another issue that Carolyn Canfield raises is patient-centered care. She says, "Patients have the answers." By this she means that the patient voice needs to be much stronger in health care in order to provide the guidance that healthcare professionals need to be sure they are providing the correct treatment to achieve the outcome desired by each patient.

Ms. Canfield believes that the design of the healthcare system inevitably leads to practitioner burnout. She believes that the fragmentation of the healthcare system impedes a sense of meaning in work by preventing practitioners from seeing the outcomes of their interactions with patients, their role in helping and healing in the lives of patients and families.

Finally, Carolyn Canfield says that this matters because health care is all about relationships. She feels that trust is betrayed when high-quality care is expected but not provided, when patient well-being is treated as subordinate to medical specialty, when no one takes responsibility for patient outcome, and when unexpected adverse outcomes are not valued as opportunities for improvement (Canfield, 2012).

Questions

1. Where do you think the system failed Nick Francis?

2. Have you witnessed fragmentation in the healthcare system? How do you think it might prevent a patient from receiving optimal care? What do you think could be done to prevent fragmentation and the problems that might arise from it?

3. How can we learn to recognize and correct care failures from fragmentation, as distinct from medical error?

4. Do you agree that the lack of patient voice is an issue in health care? Research the ways that patients are becoming involved in the design, governance, and delivery of health care. Which ways do you see as most effective?

5. What problems do you see with our current method of charting, and what do you think the individual healthcare practitioner can do about it?

6. Do you feel that more coherence in patient treatment would improve workplace satisfaction?

7. Do you agree that health care is about relationships? What sorts of actions do you think can erode trust between patient and provider, and how can these be avoided? What behaviors build trust in healthcare relationships?

8. Which of the core competencies for the health professions are most relevant for this case? Why?

References

Burningham, Z., Hashibe, M., Spector, L., & Schiffman, J. D. (2012). The epidemiology of sarcoma. *Clinical Sarcoma Research, 2*(1), 14.

Canfield, C. (2012). It's a matter of trust: A framework for patient harm. Report to the Western Canada CEOs Patient Safety Working Group. Unpublished manuscript.

Canfield, C. (2013). Resilience and reliability with the patient in the centre. Resilience Healthcare Learning Network. Available at: http://resiliencehealthcarelearningnetwork.ca/blog/resilience-and-reliability-with-the-patient-in-the-centre

Accidental Fall in a Hospital

The Story of Colin Lake (Australia)

Janet Long

Editors' Note

Accidental falls among hospital inpatients in New South Wales (NSW), Australia, are the most common adverse events in hospitals, making up a third of reported incidents (Clinical Excellence Commission and NSW Department of Health, 2010). The estimated rate of 3.88 falls per 1000 occupied bed days in NSW is similar to hospital fall rates from other countries, which range from 2.3–7.0 falls per 1000 bed days (Hitcho et al., 2004). Fischer and colleagues (2005) found that 3–10% of falls in the hospital result in an injury or fracture; others found injury rates as high as 30% (Clinical Excellence Commission and NSW Department of Health, 2010; Morse, Prowse, Morrow, & Federspeil, 1985). Physical injury and psychological damage, such as loss of confidence, are often a result, and staff can feel guilty and distressed by a perceived lack of care.

LEARNING OBJECTIVES

After completing this case study, you will be able to:

1. List patient factors that contribute to falls in the hospital setting.

2. Discuss hospital environmental and human factors that may contribute to falls (e.g., poor lighting).

3. Discuss the effectiveness of risk assessment tools for falls.

4. Consider other factors for falls that could be included in standard risk assessment tools.

5. Develop strategies for ensuring all staff are aware of the risk status for patient falls.

Background

Colin Lake was a 53-year-old business man who presented to a Sydney hospital emergency department one Friday evening with a unilateral, painful red eye. Colin used daily disposable contact lenses and reported that his right eye had been sore for 2 days. He had not removed his lens periodically as required throughout this time, thinking that taking his lenses off and on might make it worse. He presented with a bad headache and was unable to focus on his computer screen. Both contact lenses were removed and sent for culture and sensitivity.

On examination, his affected right eye appeared injected (blood-shot) and his cornea was cloudy with a central corneal ulcer that measured 2 mm by 3 mm. The visual acuity in his unaffected left eye was 6/60, but he was unable to see the chart with his right eye and was scored as "can count fingers at 1 meter." Colin admitted that he was not as careful with his contact lenses as he knew he should be, often neglecting to wash his hands before inserting them and exceeding the recommended usage time. Colin had no previous medical history but was overweight and admitted to feeling stressed after a recent acrimonious divorce.

Colin's Hospital Stay

Colin was admitted to the eye ward and was placed in a single-bed room. He was given 1 gram of Paracetamol for analgesia and commenced on a regime of intensive topical therapy consisting of Gentamicin 1% eye drops every hour, Cephalothin 1% eye drops every hour, and Homatropine 2% eye drops four times a day. Because Gentamicin and Cephalothin are known to form a precipitate in the eye if mixed together, the drops were given 30 minutes apart. Eye drops were continued at this half hourly frequency throughout Friday night, Saturday, and Saturday night. Colin was told that the ulcer needed to be treated intensively to prevent any further scarring, because the ulcer was right in the center of his cornea. Corneal damage that penetrates deeper than the superficial epithelial layer of cells, which was the case with the ulcer, results in a milky opacity that it is not possible to see through.

Colin was significantly myopic (short-sighted) but had left his prescription eyeglasses at home. However, he could see well enough to shower and eat his meals. The rest of the time he rested or listened to the radio. The nurses dimmed the lights and pulled the blinds down over the window during the day to ease his sensitivity to light (photophobia).

On Sunday morning his eye was reassessed by the ophthalmic medical resident and the drops reduced in frequency to hourly from 6:00 a.m. to 10:00 p.m. only. In spite of this improvement and an easing of the regime, Colin became increasingly annoyed and irritable with the nurses and kitchen staff, complaining about the constant interruptions of his rest, the "terrible food," and that he "couldn't get a decent coffee." One of the nurses suggested he ask his family to bring him some food more to his liking but Colin replied angrily, "I don't have any friends or family left after the divorce." He went on to say that he "felt like a leper" stuck in the side room. The nurse explained that Colin was not in isolation from the world but only from other vulnerable patients who had recently undergone eye surgery. There was no reason why he could not go downstairs to the foyer where there was a news kiosk and a coffee shop. He politely asked the nurse if she would go down and buy him a cappuccino, but she was unable to go due to work demands. So, in spite of his extreme fatigue, Colin decided that he would go and buy a coffee himself. He accepted a pair of sunglasses that the nurse offered to protect his sensitive eyes and set off for the elevator.

Colin purchased his coffee and then walked out the main entrance, intending to sit on a seat on the other side of the access road. He caught his foot on the curb and fell hard onto his outstretched right hand, injuring his right wrist, bruising both knees, and jarring his spine. He said later that he had not seen the curb at all. An x-ray of his right wrist showed a scaphoid fracture, and his hand was immobilized in a short arm thumb spica cast. The soft tissue damage to his back was treated with ice packs and topical Diclonfenac gel.

Conclusion

Colin's corneal ulcer resolved fully over the next 3 days, and the ophthalmic specialist was happy for him to continue the eye drop therapy at home; however, he was not able to self-administer his eye drops due to the plaster cast on his dominant hand. After a delay of an extra day in hospital, Colin arranged to stay with a work colleague who was able to instill the drops.

Case Discussion

Older people are clearly more vulnerable to falling than younger people, and age is considered a significant risk factor for falls. It is estimated that 26% of those older than 65 years in NSW experienced at least one fall per year in 2009 (Population Health Division, 2010). Most fall prevention risk management strategies in hospitals are targeted at the 65 and older age group; however, studies that analyze actual falls show that younger people are vulnerable, too (Hitcho et al., 2004).

Risk factors for falls in the hospital setting include gait instability, agitated confusion, urinary incontinence or frequency, a previous history of falling, and psychotropic medication (Cameron et al., 2012). Other factors that have been identified include conditions such as vertigo, being an amputee, sleep disturbance, being treated on an antihypertensive medication, and even the type of flooring

(Vieira, Freund-Heritage, & da Costa, 2011). Poor vision has also been strongly associated with an increased risk of falls among older adults (Ivers, Cumming, Mitchell, & Attebo, 1998).

Colin's hospital stay was lengthened and complicated by his fall. Because Colin's dominant hand was immobilized, on discharge he was not able to manage his eye drop therapy independently.

Considering the series of events that led to Colin's fall, it becomes apparent that there are three major issues that contributed: his poor vision, his fatigue, and that he was considered as having a very low risk of falling.

Poor Vision

Colin stated that he fell as a direct result of not being able to see the curb, and he was documented as having low vision. Three issues contributed to this poor vision: the corneal ulcer, myopia (short-sightedness), and the constant dilated right pupil due to the homatropine.

The centrally placed ulcer and swelling of the cornea had significantly compromised his sight on that side. A visual acuity of "count fingers at 1 meter" means that Colin could only distinguish how many fingers the nurse held up if her hand was brought as close as a meter from his eye. His depth perception was also affected by monocular or uneven bilateral vision, so even if Colin had seen the curb he may well have underestimated its distance and position relative to his foot.

People with normal vision often underestimate the impact of myopia on their ability to navigate obstacles safely in an unfamiliar environment. The visual acuity measurement of 6/60 in his unaffected eye meant that while he remained without his prescription glasses or contact lenses he actually fit the criteria of legal blindness. He would have been unable to see people's faces or pictures on the television clearly, and certainly would have been challenged to see the edge of the curb as he tried to cross the road.

The pain of corneal infection and inflammation is caused by spasms of the iris, resulting in photophobia. Homatropine is given by eye drop to rest the iris by fully dilating it; however, it can make the eye more vulnerable to uncomfortable light glare. The sunglasses that the nurse had provided, although effective at shielding the light, limited his vision further. Another issue was the curb itself. Low vision advocates recommend that changes in the ground level, such as steps or curbs, be painted in a contrasting color or pattern to make them more prominent. A bright yellow edge to the curb could have made it easier for Colin to see and thus avoid falling.

Fatigue

The fall occurred after 48 hours of continuous half hourly eye drop therapy. When Colin arrived at the hospital he admitted to feeling stressed and fatigued. The subsequent hospital treatment of intensive eye drop therapy had exacerbated this by constantly interrupting Colin's sleep and attempts to rest during the day. As a result, he was irritable and fatigued, and therefore more prone to accidents. Colin's isolation in a single room and his separation from family and friends, likely contributed to sense of anxiety and stress.

Risk Assessment

The accident happened outside the main entrance to the hospital. Colin was not accompanied there, because the nurse caring for him had judged him safe to ambulate alone; that is, he was deemed a low falls risk. In addition, the nurse was unavailable to go with him, and no relative or friend was available to escort him. At the time of Colin's admission there was no policy regarding the need to accompany patients being treated that leave the ward. Nurses used their clinical judgment to decide on each case individually.

Formal falls risk assessment tools are used routinely on most hospital wards (e.g., STRATIFY; Papaioannou et al., 2004; Perell et al., 2001) for all elderly patients and for younger patients. The eye ward used a risk assessment tool (similar to the one shown in **Figure 10-1**) on admission to the ward; however, Colin was not formally assessed, either because he was considered in good general health or "too young." If we apply the scoring criteria of the tool in Figure 10.1 to Colin's case, he would have been shown to have a low falls risk measure, scoring 1 for item 3, on vision, and a score of 0 for all the other items. This was in line with the assessment made by Colin's nurse as being a low falls risk. Hitcho and colleagues (2004) showed that 42% of patients who fell in an acute hospital setting had been formally assessed as having a low falls risk. This begs the question of whether risk assessment tools are effective in screening patients at risk. One large study involving 1124 residents from German nursing homes showed that the nurses' clinical judgment of patient falls risk was as accurate as predictions using risk assessment tools (Meyer, Köpke, Haastert, & Mühlhauser, 2009).

However, the usefulness of falls risk assessment tools is strongly defended for acute care patients (Perell et al., 2001). Tools allow a formal, documented assessment of factors known to be involved in the majority of falls, such as confusion and nocturia (Papaioannou et al., 2004). Interventions such as more frequent toileting and closer supervision of activities can then be planned and implemented. However, studies such as that by Hitcho et al. (2004) suggest that other factors not included in the tools may need to be considered, especially in younger patients. For example, Colin lost his vision quite suddenly and had little time to adapt to this disability. His risk cannot be compared to someone who has had poor vision for a number of years. Likewise, although Colin was not formally assessed as confused, disorientated, or anxious for item 2 on the assessment tool, he was extremely fatigued, and this may well have affected his ability to safely negotiate hazards.

Item	Falls Risk Screening Assessment	Value		Score
1. History of falls	Did the patient present to hospital with a fall or have they fallen since admission? No ☐ Yes ☐	Yes to any = 6		
	If not, has the patient fallen within the last 2 months? No ☐ Yes ☐			
2. Mental Status	Is the patient confused (i.e. unable to make purposeful decisions, disorganised thinking and memory impairment) No ☐ Yes ☐	Yes to any = 14		
	Is the patient disorientated (i.e. lacking awareness, being mistaken about time, place or person) No ☐ Yes ☐			
	Is the patient agitated (i.e. fearful affect, frequent movements and anxious)? No ☐ Yes ☐			
3. Vision	Does the patient require eyeglasses continually? No ☐ Yes ☐	Yes to any = 1		
	Does the patient report blurred vision? No ☐ Yes ☐			
	Does the patient have glaucoma, cataracts or macular degeneration? No ☐ Yes ☐			
4. Toileting	Are there any alterations in urination (i.e. frequency urgency, incontinence, nocturia)? No ☐ Yes ☐	Yes = 2		
5. Transfer score (TS) [means from bed to chair and back]	☐ Independent—use of aids to be independent is allowed	0	Add transfer score (TS) and mobility score (MS). If TS + MS between 0–2 then score = 0. If TS + MS between 3–6 then score = 7.	
	☐ Minor help—one person easily or needs supervision for safety	1		
	☐ Major help—one strong skilled helper or two normal people; physically can sit	2		
	☐ Unable no sitting balance; mechanical lifter required	3		
6. Mobility score (MS)	☐ Independent (but may use aid—e.g. cane)	0		
	☐ Walks with help of one person (verbal or physical)	1		
	☐ Wheelchair independent including corners etc	2		
	☐ Immobile	3		
Action: Total the score and follow risk recommendations according to level of risk (As validated tool, patient is at risk if total score ≥9)		0–5 Low risk 6–16 Medium risk 17–30 High risk		Total Score

Figure 10-1. Ontario Modified Stratified (Sydney Scoring) Falls Risk Screening Tool

Reproduced from the Sydney South West Area Health Service Policy Directive: SSW_PD2009_007 "Fall Injury Prevention and Management in Acute Settings," Attachment 1. Available from: www.sswahs.nsw.gov.au/pdf/policy/pd2009007.pdf.

The recommendations to care givers on the eye ward after this event were that all patients be assessed for their falls risk on admission and that all patients on intensive eye drop therapies be considered at high falls risk due to the fatigue and anxiety that often accompanies the taxing medication regime. It was further recommended that high-risk patients not leave the ward without an escort.

Interventions for patients assessed as having a high risk of falls in acute settings have met with variable success. Most studies use falls as their outcome measure, so this may miss most of the high-risk patients who do not fall. A Cochrane Review of falls interventions concluded that multifactorial interventions for older patients admitted to acute hospital wards may be the most beneficial in preventing falls (Cameron et al., 2012). However evidence was not strong, and many studies were excluded because they did not report on standard measures. The interventions considered were such things as medication review by a pharmacist to minimize drugs associated with falling, education of ancillary staff, exercise programs by physiotherapists, and scheduled toileting. These interventions had mixed success and were often setting-specific: an intervention appropriate to the orthopedic ward, for example, may be quite inappropriate for the eye ward.

Colin's story underscores that falls can happen to any patient, and that good general health and a relatively young age should not keep these patients from proper risk assessment. Falls risk assessment tools can provide a documented and formal consideration of the most common risk factors but should be combined with the clinician's expertise and knowledge of the patient and the setting-specific risks.

Questions

1. Keeping people safe from falls and allowing patients to be independent and self-reliant are sometimes conflicting goals. Should all patients be accompanied when leaving the ward?

2. The level of falls risk is usually documented in the medical record or may come up as an alert on electronic medical records. Some wards consider this inadequate and instead have a system of coloured bracelets flagging risk to all staff members. Do you think this is appropriate? Under what conditions might this be useful? When might it be considered intrusive?

3. Intensive eye drop therapy is always reviewed daily and dosage frequency decreased as soon as the threat to vision has been controlled, but it remains a demanding regime for the patients and staff constantly having their sleep and rest interrupted. Cases of extreme confusion and even psychosis have been reported by patients in high-dependency units where noise, bright lights, and around-the-clock and frequent interventions can severely impact patients. The eye ward now considers this a flag for increased falls risk. Are there other types of treatment regimes that should be considered in a falls risk assessment?

4. Poor vision is considered an invisible condition as the extent of impairment is not immediately obvious. Colin's ability to navigate safely around his room and attend to his activities of daily living (ADLs) may have misled the nurses forgetting his uncorrected myopia and overestimating his ability to go safely unaccompanied downstairs. What strategies could ensure prescription glasses are worn, if needed?

5. Some wards have implemented a very successful program of patient "watchers"; volunteers who provide extra supervision for confused patients at high risk of falling. They do not take part in actual patient care but can alert staff to the patient's increased agitation or attempts at unassisted walking or getting out of bed. This approach replaces the former reliance on keeping bed rails up and physical or chemical restraints, which can actually increase the risk of injury. What other

ideas for increasing supervision and assistance could be implemented on a ward?

6. Which of the core competencies for health professions are most relevant for this case? Why?

References

Cameron, I. D., Gillespie, L. D., Robertson, M. C., Murray, G. R., Hill, K. D., Cumming, R. G., & Kerse, N. (2012). Interventions for preventing falls in older people in care facilities and hospitals. Cochrane Database of Systematic Reviews, 12. doi: 10.1002/14651858. CD005465.pub3

Clinical Excellence Commission and NSW Department of Health. (2010). Clinical incident management in the NSW public health system 2009: January to June. Sydney: Clinical Excellence Commission and NSW Department of Health.

Fischer, I., Krauss, M., Dunagan, W. C., Birge, S., Hitcho, E., Johnson, S., . . . Fraser, V. (2005). Patterns and predictors of inpatient falls and fall-related injuries in a large academic hospital. *Infection Control and Hospital Epidemiology*, *26*(10), 822–827.

Hitcho, E. B., Krauss, M. J., Birge, S., Claiborne Dunagan, W., Fischer, I., Johnson, S., . . . Fraser, V. J. (2004). Characteristics and circumstances of falls in a hospital setting. *Journal of General Internal Medicine*, *19*(7), 732-739.

Ivers, R. Q., Cumming, R. G., Mitchell, P., & Attebo, K. (1998). Visual impairment and falls in older adults: The Blue Mountains Eye Study. *Journal of the American Geriatrics Society*, *46*(1), 58–64.

Meyer, G., Köpke, S., Haastert, B., & Mühlhauser, I. (2009). Comparison of a fall risk assessment tool with nurses' judgement alone: a cluster-randomised controlled trial. *Age and Ageing*, *38*(4), 417–423.

Morse, J., Prowse, M., Morrow, N., & Federspeil, G. (1985). A retrospective analysis of patient falls. *Canadian Journal of Public Health*, *76*(2), 116–118.

Papaioannou, A., Parkinson, W., Cook, R., Ferko, N., Coker, E., & Adachi, J. (2004). Prediction of falls using a risk assessment tool in the acute care setting. *BMC Medicine*, *2*(1), 1.

Perell, K. L., Nelson, A., Goldman, R. L., Luther, S. L., Prieto-Lewis, N., & Rubenstein, L. Z. (2001). Fall risk assessment measures: An analytic review. *The Journals of Gerontology Series A: Biological Sciences and Medical Sciences, 56*(12), M761–M766.

Population Health Division. (2010). New South Wales Fall Prevention Baseline Survey 2009. Sydney: NSW Department of Health.

Vieira, E., Freund-Heritage, R., & da Costa, B. (2011). Risk factors for geriatric patient falls in rehabilitation hospital settings: A systematic review. *Clinical Rehabilitation, 25*(9), 788–799.

Interpersonal and Communication Skills

Healthcare professionals must be able to demonstrate interpersonal and communication skills that result in the effective exchange of information and collaboration with patients, their families, and health professionals. Specific competencies within the Interprofessional and Communication Skills domain are to:

- Communicate effectively with patients, families, and the public, as appropriate, across a broad range of socioeconomic and cultural backgrounds.
- Communicate effectively with colleagues within one's profession or specialty, other health professionals, and health-related agencies.
- Work effectively with others as a member or leader of a healthcare team or other professional group.
- Act in a consultative role to other health professionals.
- Maintain comprehensive, timely, and legible medical records.
- Demonstrate sensitivity, honesty, and compassion in difficult conversations, including those about death, end of life, adverse events, bad news, disclosure of errors, and other sensitive topics.

- Demonstrate insight and understanding about emotions and human responses to emotions that allow one to develop and manage.

Section 4 starts with Case 11, "Not Considered a Partner: A Mother's Story of a Tonsillectomy Gone Wrong," written by Tanya Lord. In 1999, Tanya's son, Noah, was 4 years old when an otolaryngologist recommended that he have a tonsillectomy and adenoidectomy. Tanya Lord tells the story of Noah's surgery and postoperative death.

Case 12, "Lost: A Patient's Search for Answers for Intractable Pain," tells the story of Claudine Goze-Weber, a retired government worker living in southeastern France, who was left in chronic pain from a failed surgical procedure for chronic back pain. This case involves a lack of informed consent and a search for answers from the medical establishment. Claudine's life was changed by her decision to have surgery, based on information she had read on the Internet.

In Case 13, "The Silence of the Hospital: Lessons on Supporting Patients and Staff After an Adverse Event," Linda Kenny tells the story of the surgery that was planned for her right ankle replacement. The surgery did not proceed as planned when the popliteal fossa block, in which bupivacaine was supposed to be injected into a nerve in the back of her knee to numb the lower leg and ankle, was injected into a blood vessel instead of the nerve. Linda had a seizure followed by a cardiac arrest. Linda focuses the case on the aftermath of the adverse event, in which the hospital failed to provide adequate support to Linda or to the providers involved in the case.

As in other sections of the book, we caution the reader that these cases are complex and include elements of other competencies as well. As you read the cases, it is helpful to think about the other competencies that are relevant. (Refer to the full list of competencies in the appendix.)

Not Considered a Partner: A Mother's Story of a Tonsillectomy Gone Wrong

The Story of Noah Lord (United States)

Tanya Lord

Editors' Note

More than 500,000 tonsillectomies are performed each year on children in the United States, most commonly for sleep-disordered breathing and recurrent throat infections. Most parents regard tonsillectomies as free of risk to their children's well-being; however, tonsillectomies can be risky, with bleeding and vomiting accompanied by dehydration as the most serious complications causing a return of children to the hospital after a tonsillectomy (Mahant et al., 2014). Substantial variation exists in the quality of care for routine tonsillectomy across the United States. Significant variation in care processes and outcomes continues today.

Tanya Lord tells the story of her 4-year-old son, Noah, who died in 1999 following a tonsillectomy and adenoidectomy.

LEARNING OBJECTIVES

After completing this case study, you will be able to:

1. Outline the system issues that led to Noah's death.
2. Discuss how to address the problem of fragmentation in health care.

3. Create a strategy to meaningfully partner with patients and families to achieve high-quality health care.

4. Discuss tools for analysis and disclosure of adverse events in hospitals.

Noah's Story

Noah was born in 1995 and suffered from continual ear infections as an infant. When he was 1 year old, his hearing was evaluated because he was not babbling and talking the way one would expect from a 1-year-old child. The ear infections and chronic fluid behind his ears caused speech delays because he could not hear correctly. When Noah was 2 years old, he had a set of special ear tubes placed in his ears to relieve the ear infections. Noah's speech rapidly improved. In 1999, when Noah was 4, we moved from Boston to New Jersey, and Noah's new ear, nose, and throat (ENT) specialist recommended that Noah have a tonsillectomy and adenoidectomy. (**Figure 11-1** provides an overview of Noah's care.)

The ENT doctor asked about Noah's snoring and questioned if he had obstructive sleep apnea (OSA). While living in Boston, we had recorded Noah's sleeping pattern and noises, and we were confident that Noah did not have OSA. The week before his scheduled surgery I asked the ENT if it were possible to remove the adenoids and leave the tonsils. He responded that there was an option to do that, but that he was pretty sure that in 6 months Noah would need to have the tonsils removed and that it would be cruel to put Noah under anesthesia twice in 1 year. We agreed to the surgery to remove both the tonsils and the adenoids, because the ENT seemed confident that this was the right decision.

The Surgery and Postsurgical Events

Noah underwent surgery on a Friday morning. Following the surgery we were told that he had done fine in the surgery and had come out of anesthesia well, but he was not eating or drinking. They had told me earlier that he would be discharged once he had drunk

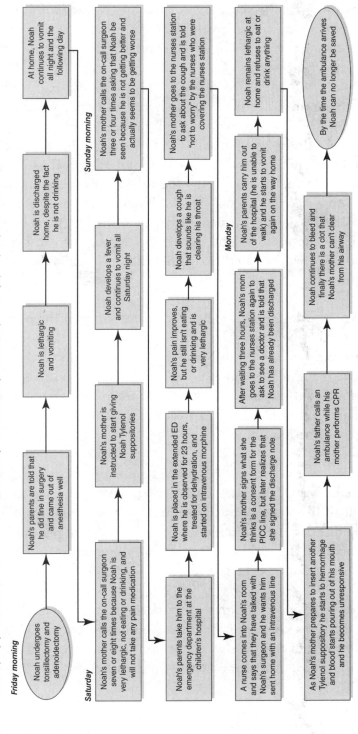

Noah Lord's Story – "Just a Routine Tonsillectomy"

Noah suffered from continual ear infections as an infant. When he was one year old, his hearing was evaluated because he was not babbling and talking the way one would expect from a child his age. The ear infections and chronic fluid behind his ears had caused speech delays because he wasn't hearing correctly. When Noah was two years old, he had a set of tubes put in his ears that relieved the ear infections and his speech improved. When Noah was four, his family moved from Boston to New Jersey, and Noah's new ear, nose, and throat (ENT) specialist recommended that Noah have a tonsillectomy and adenoidectomy. This is the story of his surgery and postoperative death.

Figure 11-1. Noah's Story

145

something, but he never drank anything. He was vomiting, and they attributed that to the anesthesia. He was pretty lethargic and miserable, which they said was to be expected. They discharged Noah, and we were happy to go home.

Noah continued to throw up at home all Friday night and the following day. On Saturday, I called the on-call surgeon several times just because he was becoming very lethargic, he was not eating or drinking anything, and he would not take any oral pain medication. I was told that it was likely due to the anesthesia combined with his level of pain. They suggested Tylenol suppositories because he would not take any medication orally. Although Noah was given the Tylenol suppositories, he started developing a fever. He continued to throw up all night. He was not recovering like they said that he would.

On Sunday morning, I called the on-call surgeon three or four times asking that Noah be seen because he was not getting any better and seemed to be quite a bit worse. We took Noah to the emergency department at the children's hospital. He was not admitted to the hospital, but was observed for 23 hours in the extended emergency department (ED). He was treated for dehydration and started on intravenous morphine.

His pain improved, but he still was not eating or drinking the entire time he was in the emergency department. They tried to entice him with slushies and popsicles—anything they could think of, but he wouldn't eat anything. He was extremely lethargic and I was concerned, but they told me that the morphine was making him groggy and it was to be expected.

Noah developed a cough that sounded like he was clearing his throat all the time. I went to the nurses' station to ask if this was normal and was told that this was okay and "not to worry." They were not ED nurses but covering nurses from obstetrics.

While in the ED we saw a variety of different surgeons and nurses but were never really sure who was in charge as they were not identified and often neglected to introduce themselves by name. The surgeon who performed Noah's surgery consulted by phone—and never showed up to examine Noah.

At one time, a woman came in and I grabbed her by the wrist and pulled her over to the bedside and I said, "He really is not doing well." I asked the woman to just look at him, to help me, and she responded, "I am really sorry, but I am just here to take the dirty laundry." At one point an older gentleman poked his head in and said, "How's it going in here?" I responded automatically, "Okay," and then the man disappeared. I found out later that he was the emergency room attending physician. I met with him 10 years later, and he remembered poking his head in the room and walking away.

A nurse came in and announced that they had talked to Noah's surgeon and that he wanted him sent home with an intravenous line (PICC line) so he would be able to receive fluids at home. A visiting nurse would come to our home during the evening so Noah would sleep with an IV.

The nurse handed me a paper to sign and I signed it. This was Monday morning following Noah's surgery on Friday. I was so exhausted that I just signed the paper without looking at it. The nurse left the room, and I waited for about 3 to 4 hours without anyone coming into the room. So I went to the nursing station again and I told them that I really wanted to talk to a doctor. The nurses' response was, "You can't talk to a doctor; you have been discharged." This was the first time that I realized that the paper I had signed was his discharge paper. I told them that I still really needed to talk to a doctor and I did not feel comfortable taking Noah home. The nurse told me, "There is nothing we can do." I did not want to go home because I knew it was not the right thing to do, but I also did not know how to push back and did not know what to say.

We carried him out of the hospital and Noah started vomiting again during the drive home. When we got home we tried to entice him to eat or drink but he wouldn't. He remained lethargic. We continued to give him Tylenol suppositories, and when it was time for another dose, I laid him on the bathroom floor to insert the suppository. While lying on the floor as I put his pull-up on he sat up and he looked at me and he said, "Mommy," and then he started to hemorrhage. Blood came pouring out of his mouth and out of his nose and he stopped breathing. I had trained to be a lifeguard, so I knew CPR and I was able to resuscitate him three different times with some responsiveness and a pulse. My husband was upstairs and I was screaming at him, "Call an ambulance." While the ambulance was on their way they were trying to tell me what to do and he just kept bleeding. There was finally a clot that I could not clear from his airway and he died before the ambulance arrived. When they arrived there was nothing else they could do.

After Noah's death, the hospital stopped responding to our requests for information. The surgeon talked to us for a little while, but he became more and more frustrated with talking to me. At one point he said, "I do not understand what happened to your son and if I do not understand it then you're certainly never going to understand it." It seemed like the only way to get information about the case and the decisions that led to Noah's death was to file a lawsuit. If they had just engaged us and responded honestly to our questions, allowed us talk to the providers that treated Noah, and let us know that they were looking into the issues around our son's death, then it would have saved us a lot of heartache and definitely saved them a lawsuit.

Ten years later, the academic medical center where Noah received his care asked me to present Noah's case to medical students. I thought if I was going to tell his story then I wanted all who were involved, including the hospital, to know. I sent them my presentation and wanted them to know what I was doing. They invited me back to spend a day meeting with the different providers who had taken care of Noah and some who were new. They recognized and admitted to some of the problems that they had had in the emergency department. This meeting was good, but it was just 10 years too late.

Conclusion

I went to graduate school and completed a master's degree in public health, which focused on medical error as a threat to public health. I realized that there was a lot of work to be done to reduce harm from medical error. I completed the master's degree and continued into a PhD program motivated by a desire to help others who had undergone a similar situation.

In working with other bereaved parents I realized how difficult it is to find help and to find the right kind of support to navigate the system. Many hospitals do not have bereavement groups. When people are grieving or are newly bereaved they do not have the capacity to find the resources that are available. My husband and I developed a Grief Toolbox (https://thegrieftoolbox.com), which is an online resource to bring different bereavement practices and aids to help other people who have similar losses. In this situation the most helpful people are those who have experienced a similar loss. We are working on *Walking Through Grief*, which is an educational video series using the stories and the words from people who are bereaved.

Case Discussion

Noah's story is a classic example of a cascading series of systems issues that led to patient harm and to his death. There was not a single gross error or gross negligence. At multiple points things could have gone differently, starting with the decision to have a tonsillectomy.

About 530,000 tonsillectomies are now performed each year on children in the United States. As in Noah's case, tonsillectomy is often combined with adenoidectomy in an operation called an adenotonsillectomy. Together, tonsillectomy and adenotonsillectomy make up the second most common pediatric surgery in the United States, exceeded only by myringotomy, or placement of ear tubes to relieve recurrent ear infections, a procedure that Noah also underwent. There is substantial disagreement over the effectiveness and appropriateness of tonsillectomy, and the wide variation in frequency appears to be related to differences in clinical practice rather than to clinical need (Baugh et al., 2011). For most of the twentieth century, tonsillectomy to help prevent recurrent throat infections was the most widely performed surgical procedure in the United States. Tonsillectomy rates declined after doubts were raised over its effectiveness for that purpose. In recent decades, rates of tonsillectomy, and particularly adenotonsillectomy, have risen again as they have gained currency as a treatment for sleep-disordered breathing, a term comprising a spectrum of disorders ranging from snoring to obstructive sleep apnea. In 2005, 77% of all tonsillectomies and adenotonsillectomies were done for sleep-disordered breathing (Erickson et al., 2009). Evidence-based guidelines exist for tonsillectomy, but their application is highly variable. Hospital revisits within 30 days average 7.8%, but the rate of revisit is also highly variable from institution to institution (Mahant et al., 2014).

Noah did not have sleep apnea, but there was miscommunication, and the surgeon was under the impression that Noah had sleep apnea. Noah was treated appropriately for dehydration, but no one considered that there were other possible complications. There was a breakdown in communication in the emergency department because Noah was really not "owned" by anybody, and no care provider felt accountable. The surgeon treated him as an ED patient, so he consulted by phone, and the ED staff felt like he was a surgical patient, and so he was never fully accounted for. As a result, he was not treated like a postsurgical patient, and his surgical site was never evaluated properly.

When patients and families are well informed and well educated, they can get better health care. It is difficult to partner with somebody who does not have the education or the understanding of the healthcare system. Education is needed for patients and families as well as for providers. As Noah's mother states, "I was not considered a partner in Noah's care. There was not a lot of thought given to the concerns I raised as his mother."

Questions

1. What were the barriers that prevented Noah from receiving effective care in the emergency department?

2. What communication failures were apparent in Noah's care?

3. Perform an Internet search to find the clinical practice guidelines for tonsillectomy in children.

   a. What do the guidelines recommend regarding perioperative management of children undergoing tonsillectomy?

   b. How could these guidelines have prevented Noah's harm?

4. Informed consent plays an important role in helping patients and families make good decisions. How could the informed consent process be improved in this case?

5. Would mandatory identification of healthcare providers (such as on their coats or badges, etc.), including their role and seniority, have helped in this case? How would you suggest addressing this issue?

6. Which of the core competencies for health professions are most relevant for this case? Why?

References

Baugh, R. F., Archer, S. M., Mitchell, R. B., Rosenfeld, R. M., Amin, R., Burns, J. J., . . . Patel, M. M. (2011). Clinical practice guideline: Tonsillectomy in children. *Otolaryngology—Head and Neck Surgery, 144*(1 Suppl), S1–S30.

Erickson, B. K., Larson, D. R., St Sauver, J. L., Meverden, R. A., & Orvidas, L. J. (2009). Changes in incidence and indications of tonsillectomy and adenotonsillectomy, 1970–2005. *Otolaryngology—Head and Neck Surgery, 140*(6), 894–901.

Mahant, S., Keren, R., Localio, R., Luan, X., Song, L., Shah, S. S., . . . Srivastava, R. (2014). Variation in quality of tonsillectomy perioperative care and revisit rates in children's hospitals. *Pediatrics, 133*(2), 280–288.

Lost: A Patient's Search for Answers for Intractable Pain

The Story of Claudine Goze-Weber (France)

Julie Johnson, Helen Haskell, and Paul Barach

Editors' Note

Claudine Goze-Weber's story was a long one, spanning over a decade. But after years of talking to other patients, she did not believe it was an unusual one. Claudine was a retired government worker living in southeastern France. She suffered from two disorders of the spine: arachnoiditis (inflammation of the arachnoid membrane surrounding the nerves of the spinal cord) and Tarlov cysts, cerebrospinal fluid-filled bulges in the sheath of the spinal nerves. Arachnoiditis can arise from a number of factors, including infection, reactions to chemicals or drugs, or trauma to the spine. Iatrogenic causes include back surgery and contaminated or improperly placed epidural steroids or anesthetics, as Claudine believed happened in her case. Arachnoiditis can cause debilitating pain, especially in the later stages, when scar tissue and adhesions may encapsulate and stiffen the nerves (Burton, 1978; National Institute of Neurological Disorders and Stroke, 2011).

Although their actual incidence is not known, Tarlov cysts are officially classified as a rare condition by the U.S. National Institutes of Health (Office of Rare Diseases Research, 2014). They are typically located in the sacrum, the five fused vertebrae at the base of the spine. They are usually asymptomatic and are often first seen as incidental findings on medical images of the spine. Treatment is not recommended for asymptomatic cysts. The causes of Tarlov cysts are not definitively known, but theories include inflammation, hemorrhage, trauma, and congenital origins. Asymptomatic cysts are thought sometimes to become symptomatic as a result of back trauma (Acosta, Quinones-Hinojosa, Schmidt, & Weinstein, 2003). Symptoms of Tarlov cyst disease can include lower back and leg pain, urinary incontinence, constipation, and headaches, although there is no clear way to distinguish symptoms of Tarlov cysts from those due to other causes. Cysts are known to enlarge over time, possibly leading to worsening of symptoms. Although surgical treatment is controversial, a small number of practitioners offer surgical and other interventions for symptomatic cysts, including filling the cysts with fat or fibrin glue (Long, 2011).

Claudine Goze-Weber died in June 2013. Prior to her death, she had become a significant online presence and had done much to raise the profile and improve the level of knowledge available about arachnoiditis and Tarlov cysts. It was her belief that suffering among people with these conditions was exacerbated by non-evidence-based treatments promoted over the Internet to desperate patients.

The following is taken from an interview with Claudine conducted on January 16, 2013.

LEARNING OBJECTIVES

After completing this case study, you will be able to:

1. Outline the elements of an effective informed consent process.
2. Explain ways that stereotyping can be harmful to patients.
3. Discuss strategies for encouraging patients to be informed consumers.
4. Debate the potential benefit and harm from the availability of medical information on the Internet.

Mysterious Symptoms

Prior to my original medical injury, I was a healthy and active person. I worked for the juridical team of the French National Health System, and I regularly walked and swam for recreation. That all changed in 1992, when I was given epidural anesthesia for a minor surgical procedure. As soon as the effects of the anesthesia wore off, I was overwhelmed with a horrible burning pain that was almost more than I could endure. I had never experienced such pain, even when giving birth to my two sons.

I was told that the pain was nothing to worry about. But after I went home, I began to feel tired all the time. I had severe cramps in the abdomen. I was unable to sleep, and I had terrible headaches and backaches. All the doctors I saw told me my symptoms were related to the premenopausal period. This went on for 9 years. Then in the fall of 2001 I began to have problems with my balance. At the end of November 2001, I had a serious fall and hit my back on the edge of the stairs. I could not walk and I was in horrible pain. When I went to the hospital, the MRI showed advanced arachnoiditis, with scar tissue calcified from the second to the fifth lumbar vertebra. It also showed seven Tarlov cysts in the sacral vertebrae at the base of the spinal column.

At the time there was a major strike by the medical profession in France. I was treated in emergency rooms, and I never saw the same doctor twice. They were overbooked; the ones who were working had too much to do, and they knew I was not going to be their patient. I was searching for an answer, a simple answer, and I went from one doctor to another, with nobody telling me what it was about. I think now that they did not want to tell me that there was nothing they could do to improve my condition.

I met with many specialists. They surely knew, but nobody told me. They said, "Oh, I don't know. I don't know. Don't do anything." But nobody told me why. Nobody explained to me, "You know, you have nerve fiber damage and this can't be reversed. This is something you can't do anything for. You are going to have this condition. You are going to have pain. But it is not dangerous. You can go on living. And if you do some exercises you are maybe going to be better, at least for part of the day."

I met a neurosurgeon who told me, "Yes, you have Tarlov cysts, but it's better not to touch them." I searched online for information about Tarlov cysts and found only websites and forums telling of surgery to treat them. And reading on the forums of wonderful surgeries by wonderful people who could treat these cysts, in my head I thought, "The doctors here just don't want to help me." The people on the forums, some of whom were in the medical profession, said, "Yes, you need surgery." I trusted them, because I didn't know otherwise. I sought another neurosurgeon and I found one who told me, "Oh, yes, I can do the surgery." I had no idea that it would not help me.

He did not explain that the Tarlov cyst procedure of fat injection was a major back surgery. He let me think that it was a shot, like the fluoroscopy shot that had been used to assess my neuronal damage. But it is a serious operation. They open the sacrum. They make a hole. They do a laminectomy. They open the back, they open the muscle, they go to the fat; they take some fat and plug it in the cyst. They say it is to relieve pressure, but they take out the spinal fluid, which is very light, and instead put in fat or glue, which has more weight. Now that I have learned more about it, the surgery does not make much sense to me.

Surgical Consequences

I had surgery on August 8, 2002, and I have been in severe pain most of the time since. Before the surgery, I had Tarlov cysts, but my spine was not cut; my muscles were not cut. I did not have spinal instability, which is excessive movement between the vertebrae. The surgery made me worse because of the mechanical consequences of cutting the muscle, creating scar tissue, and so on. I lost my job because of the disability. Worst of all, because I have an allergy to morphine and opioid medications, I can't treat the pain with medication. I have almost no pain management, except some techniques for deep relaxation.

When I called the surgeon after the operation, he said, "You know, I am not a miracle man. If I had told you about the seriousness of the operation, you wouldn't have gone." He told me that he did not tell me because he did not want me to worry and to refuse to have surgery. The feeling of being misled, of having life-changing surgery without my consent, still upsets me, so much that I am often very anxious and not far from deep depression.

In 2003, I sent my files to four different specialists, without any other comment than the description of my symptoms and medical history. The four reports came back with similar conclusions: calcified arachnoiditis that could only be due to epidural anesthesia, scar tissue at the site of the Tarlov cyst surgery, plus severe spine instability due to the fact that main ligaments had been cut. Only a third of the sacrum bone remains, and a large piece of it is now encysted in the middle of a mix of muscle and nerve scar tissue. There is scar tissue at each level of the sacral vertebrae.

I also had an unexpected problem with my family doctor. He became annoyed and upset with me and acted as though he did not believe that my symptoms were real. It was awful. He told my husband, "She needs to go to a psychologist or to a psychiatric hospital." As I am allergic to painkillers, I was going regularly to a professor of pain management who was teaching me to deal with pain using deep relaxation techniques. This doctor was also a psychiatrist. I gave her the letter the family doctor had written about my needing to go to a psychiatric hospital and asked her opinion. She took the letter, she made a copy, she tore it in two, and she said, "You go on with your life, and we are going to go on and do the pain management." This relieved me, because I no longer had any confidence in myself. I was completely lost.

Later when I went for the disability test I had to go before both a physical medical team and a psychiatric medical team. I spent 2 hours in front of the director of the psychiatric hospital, and he told me, "Yes, you are disabled." He did not think I had a psychiatric problem.

It was very odd, very strange. By the end of an experience like that you no longer know who you are, what you are, and what is wrong or not wrong with you.

In 2009 I had a detailed laser image that showed exactly where the main damage was. It was not from the Tarlov cysts. It was higher up, at the lumbar level where my back was hit by the edge of the stair when I fell down the stairs. If I had been told this immediately—and I believe they could have told me immediately—I would not have had the surgery.

Later I had to copy my file for a new doctor. And rereading the file, I saw that in fact from the very beginning it was obvious that the problem was not the Tarlov cysts. I finally discovered that by myself. It was like a puzzle. I put one piece here, one other piece there, another piece there. I studied it all. I reread my MRI report and each little thing that had happened during those years. This final conclusion is the only conclusion that makes sense—not only for my story, but the story of all the patients I have met.

Conclusion

I felt that I had been led into this mistaken surgery by the information I had found on the Internet. I began to share my story and to make websites about Tarlov cysts and arachnoiditis so that people could find reliable information. I needed to understand this in order to face what had happened to me. I have a scientific and technical background, and with the help of some doctors and specialists I went back to my studies of physiology and neurology. I created a website now called *Tarlov et Arachnoïdite* (Tarlov cyst and Arachnoiditis) and began sharing with friends and colleagues from all over the world, with specialists to provide information.

I am only one voice. There are other patients online who are pushing the others to go to surgery. Those people speak very positively, and many patients want to hear about positive outcomes and want to hear that they are going to be better. And they go, as I did. You cannot tell those people about negative outcomes, because you are not trusted. I have been attacked, told I am a negative person. I have been called a fake, even though my website is certified by the HONcode of medical ethics.

People who have Tarlov cyst surgery have often been told that if they don't have the surgery they will become paralyzed. Even though there are highly qualified specialists who explain that this is not true, other specialists are not telling the patient. And you can see the result of that in the online forums. People are afraid. They do not know whom to believe.

It's a disadvantage to try to talk about medical evidence when I am not part of the medical profession. People say, "Oh, she is not a medical professional. She doesn't understand." But as I tell them, everything can be learned. Even doctors learn, even nurses learn. And what they learn, we also can learn. Of course I didn't learn by myself. I had the help of expert doctors. I had a scientific background, so it was not too difficult for me to understand. But like the doctors, I had to learn.

Case Discussion

Claudine Goze-Weber's story addresses matters of uncertainty and trust in medicine, focused on one of the most frustrating symptoms that both patients and clinicians face: chronic back pain. Chronic back pain is one of the most difficult issues in medicine. The cause is often unclear, and treatments can be risky or, as Claudine found, even questionable. Doctors worry about patients becoming addicted to pain medications. For Claudine, this was not an issue because she specifically avoided narcotic drugs, yet she still suffered the experience of not being believed and of being given a psychiatric diagnosis when she sought help for real and urgent symptoms. For Claudine, this was a tremendous and, she felt, unnecessary, emotional burden.

Claudine's is also a story of lack of informed consent and a search for answers from the medical establishment. Claudine was haunted by the fact that she was not given the information she needed to make decisions that were in line with her own preferences. She felt that she was left in the dark by doctors who were uncomfortable in relaying bad news and, even more, that she was harmed by paternalism: doctors who felt that, for her own good, they should not give her information that might cause her to worry or to make decisions they did not agree with.

Patients who do not get explanations and a sympathetic handling of their problems will not stop looking for answers. Claudine's life was clearly changed by her decision to have surgery, based on information she read on the Internet. She felt that this decision had been based on false hope offered by information that was not grounded in the evidence. She made it her life's work to try to be sure that patients with arachnoiditis and Tarlov cysts had access to reliable information, and in so doing changed the picture of how these conditions are presented to the public.

Questions

1. Research the topic of shared decision making and discuss the various options that doctors might have had in explaining a case like this one. Why do you think Claudine's doctors might not have given her the information she needed?

2. Have you seen instances of paternalism, and do you think it is a significant problem in the practice of medicine?

3. Claudine Goze-Weber described Internet forums and websites where patients were encouraged to have procedures that might not be in line with accepted medical evidence. At the same time, she strongly believed in the importance of patients doing their own research and learning about their own conditions. How do you think these two considerations can best be balanced?

4. Claudine's Tarlov cysts were discovered on images taken when she suffered pain after a fall. She came to believe that the cysts were an incidental finding and were not responsible for her symptoms. Research the interpretive problems

surrounding incidental findings in medicine. How do you think this difficult issue can best be addressed?

5. Claudine Goze-Weber described very eloquently the "lost" feeling she had when she no longer knew whether to trust her own judgment about herself. What do you think the psychological effect might be on patients who are told by a physician that the symptoms they are experiencing are not real? How do you think healthcare professionals can be more sensitive to this issue? Do you think psychiatric diagnoses are overused in this context?

6. Which of the core competencies for health professions do you think are most relevant for this case? Why?

References

Acosta, F. L., Jr., Quinones-Hinojosa, A., Schmidt, M. H., & Weinstein, P. R. (2003). Diagnosis and management of sacral Tarlov cysts. Case report and review of the literature. *Neurosurgical Focus, 15*(2), E15.

Burton, C. V. (1978). Lumbosacral arachnoiditis. *Spine (Phila Pa 1976), 3*(1), 24–30.

Long, D. (2011). About symptomatic Tarlov cysts. Available at: http://www.donlinlong.com/clinical/procedures/tarlovpatients/

National Institute of Neurological Disorders and Stroke. (2011). NINDS arachnoiditis information page. Available at: http://www.ninds.nih.gov/disorders/arachnoiditis/arachnoiditis.htm

Office of Rare Diseases Research, Genetic and Rare Diseases Information Center. (2011). Tarlov cysts. Available at: http://rarediseases.info.nih.gov/gard/9258/tarlov-cysts/resources/1

The Silence of the Hospital: Lessons on Supporting Patients and Staff After an Adverse Event

The Story of Linda Kenney (United States)

Linda Kenney

Editors' Note

Linda Kenney considered herself nearly a professional patient. Born with bilateral club feet, she had undergone 19 corrective surgeries over the course of her life. In addition, her job was in health care: she worked as an administrative assistant in an operating room in a large medical center and felt confident that she understood the system well. "I was an administrative worker, not a clinician," she says, "but I got to see amazing things."

In 1999, Linda was scheduled for her twentieth surgery, a right ankle replacement. An educated healthcare consumer, she went to the hospital with a list of things she wanted. This included a request for an attending physician as her anesthesiologist. Linda and the surgeon had decided that her anesthesia would be a popliteal fossa block, in which the numbing agent bupivacaine would be injected into a nerve in the back of her knee to numb the lower leg and ankle. Linda did not want a resident doing this procedure. A board-certified anesthesiologist named Rick van Pelt was scheduled to handle her nerve block.

On the day of the operation, Linda told her husband to go on to work until the surgery was over. But the surgery did not go forward as planned. After the anesthesiologist administered the popliteal fossa block, Linda had a seizure, followed by cardiac arrest.

The anesthesiologist had missed the nerve and accidentally injected the bupivacaine into the blood vessel instead.

Because she was in a large teaching hospital with immediate access to specialized knowledge and equipment, Linda survived her cardiac arrest, but she suffered lingering physical effects and ongoing emotional trauma. Most disturbing of all, she felt, was the hospital's failure to provide support either to her and her family or to Dr. van Pelt and the other clinicians involved. Linda tells the story of her brush with death in the hospital and her subsequent founding of the nonprofit organization MITSS—Medically Induced Trauma Support Services—whose mission is "To Support Healing and Restore Hope" to patients, families and clinicians following adverse medical events.

LEARNING OBJECTIVES

After completing this case study, you will be able to:

1. Describe the potential effects of a medical error or adverse medical event on patients, families, and health professionals.

2. Discuss elements of a strategy for disclosing adverse events and medical errors.

3. Create a strategy for supporting medically harmed patients and their families.

4. Create a strategy for supporting health professionals who have been involved in harming a patient.

A Near-Death Experience

I remember everything that happened that day before the surgery was supposed to take place. I remember rolling into the preholding area. I remember telling the anesthesiologist that I was very uncomfortable about the block. He told me not to worry, that he had done it a hundred times. He will tell you now that he has never said that again. In fact, he will tell you that when he saw the list of things I wanted, his immediate reaction was, "She is going to be a pain." Today, his thinking has changed to, "This is a patient who has some experience and we need to have a conversation before the surgery." So his practice has changed because of what happened that day.

From the beginning, I had a bad feeling about this surgery. I had signed many consent forms, but this was the first time I had looked at a form and had the word "death" pop out at me. I don't know why I felt that way, but when I think back I would say to any patient, "If you have a bad feeling, honor that feeling. It does not matter how crazy you feel, honor that bad feeling."

The last thing I remember is saying goodbye to my husband. Then we went into the preoperative holding area, and that was where they injected the block. The procedure consisted of going in past the blood vessels into the nerve. To do this they have to pull back on the needle; if there is no blood then they are sure they are into the nerve. But when the anesthesiologist pulled back on the needle there was no blood, so he put the medication in, and apparently it went into the blood vessel anyway. What they think happened was that he did not get any blood because it was a broken-down vessel. Bupivacaine is a cardiotoxic drug and within a minute I had a grand mal seizure followed by a full cardiac arrest. They called a cardiac code and started advanced cardiac life support right away, but after 15 minutes I was still unresponsive.

Luckily for me, there just happened to be a doctor there who had experience with this. He knew that the only way to save my life would be to get me onto cardiac bypass right away. Again, things were in my favor that day: there was a cardiac suite already prepared for another patient, with a cardiopulmonary bypass machine primed and ready. They bumped the other patient and within 35 minutes they had opened my chest and had me hooked up to a cardiopulmonary bypass machine so that the medication could be flushed out of my system.

My husband was not even out of the main lobby before I had the cardiac arrest. He got a phone call from the orthopedic surgeon who had stood by in horror watching the whole incident unfold. The surgeon said, "Mr. Kenney, there has been a problem with the anesthesia. We had to crack your wife's chest; you need to come in." My husband just dropped the phone and immediately returned. My husband didn't know where to go, but a woman from admitting recognized him and brought him into a room. He was left alone in a small room until somebody came to get him. I think about that now. Somebody should have been with my husband.

The anesthesiologist and orthopedic surgeon waited for a while before they came to talk to him. As soon as they opened the door my husband physically went after them. He said, "What have you done to my beautiful wife?!" The orthopedic surgeon's reply was, "It doesn't look good. We don't know what the outcome is going to be."

When I woke up I was on a ventilator in the intensive care unit. No one wanted to talk about what had happened. Someone told me I had had an allergic reaction to the anesthesia. I knew intuitively that was wrong, so right away, as I lay there in the hospital, I felt unsafe and untrusting. That was not a good mental state to be in after what I had been through. My husband did not want to leave my side and did not want anybody near me; I'm sure he was marked by the staff as a difficult family member. I found out years later that they did not ever ask him to leave. They actually changed their practice because they saw that my husband's voice helped calm me down. I was the first patient to change this practice.

I remember worrying about my children. There was no support for any of my family members. You could see that the staff felt bad for me, but nobody was talking. My orthopedic surgeon could barely look at me. I remember writing a note asking if he had replaced my ankle. He shook his head and looked down. It took me a good week to grasp that my ankle had not been replaced.

I felt abandoned. I had a rewired chest, broken ribs, and I looked as though I had been beaten up. I remember taking that first shower and having somebody wash me because I could not do it and feeling the most vulnerable I had ever felt in my life. I got my chart before I left the hospital and it said right on the front, "Allergy to PENICILLIN and BUPIVACAINE." That was the route they were going.

Alone at Home

When I left the hospital, I received instructions on caring for my incision and information about a visiting nurse. That was all. I never got a phone call. All I got was a bill. I had had many day surgeries when they would call me the next day and ask how I was doing. This time they almost killed me and I didn't even get a call.

A week after I got home I received a letter from the anesthesiologist, Dr. van Pelt. I did not know that he had tried to see me several times in the hospital, but that multiple things had stopped that from happening. In the letter he said he was sorry for what had happened and that he believed in open and honest communication. He gave me his home telephone number and cell number. I had no idea that what he was doing was so ahead of the time. My feelings at the time were that this was damage control. I filed the letter, and did not think about it for a long time.

When I got home, Christmas was coming. My kids were all still reacting to what had happened. I was trying to take care of their needs, and I was physically very limited. It was a slow recovery. At the time, I coped by focusing on being thankful to be alive and taking care of my family.

A couple of months later I was feeling better physically. My family and friends thought I had moved on, but I know today that I had not yet processed my emotions. Then, while at a wake for a 14-year-old child, I began to feel guilty. I felt guilty that I got to live and this child had died. It was like the floodgate opened, and every feeling I had been pushing down just came out. I began crying and felt as though I was never going to stop. I remember crying over folding towels. I just felt isolated and alone for months.

I needed a cortisone shot in my right ankle due to severe pain because I had not had the ankle replaced. I made an appointment to see my orthopedic surgeon. I went in and told him that I thought we should talk about what had happened. His entourage left the room and he told me what the day was like for him.

He said, "That day is burned in my memory like the birth of my children, although those were joyful occasions and this was not. Linda, you are a miracle." By that time everybody was telling me I was a miracle and I did not believe it. He said, "No, Linda, you are a miracle from God," and he began to cry.

My first reaction was, "What? What are you doing?" But then compassion came over me and I looked at him in a different light. I felt bad for him. It was the first time that anybody had showed me that they cared and that this had had an effect on them, too. As the patient, I needed this. It really made me feel better to see this reaction, but almost at once he stopped the story and would not finish. He got up, walked to the door, and left.

A few days after this meeting I called the hospital to ask if there were other patients I could talk to who had gone through this same thing. I knew I could not be the only one and I needed others to talk to. They never called me back. Months later I called my orthopedic surgeon again and asked whether he thought it would be reasonable for me to invite Dr. van Pelt for coffee. That was when I found out that Dr. van Pelt was no longer in Boston. I felt as though the floor had dropped out from under me. I thought I had missed the opportunity to ever hear the anesthesiologist's perspective and get closure on our shared event.

Luckily for me, the orthopedic surgeon was very proactive. He reached out to the head of anesthesia department, who contacted Dr. van Pelt. This ultimately led to my phone conversation with Dr. van Pelt, which was wonderful for me because I got to hear how affected he was. I felt as though I finally had gotten to hear the truth from somebody.

I was the first person who had asked him how he was doing. This struck me as so odd. Eventually I met other people who had been on the code team and all they could do was cry. I remember meeting a nursing supervisor who had been taking care of the patient next to me and I told her I often wondered how the other patients going into surgery dealt with seeing this scene unfold right in front of their eyes. She said that for the people who stayed overnight, she went up to see them in their rooms. She took it upon herself to do this all on her own.

I called the hospital and told them that I could not read the writing in the chart, but that I would like to know who everybody was on my code team because I wanted to write them a letter. It was coming up on my 1-year anniversary and I really wanted to thank them for doing their job. I knew that for them it was just their job, but I wanted to articulate how this had affected my family and me and what it meant to us. I never got a phone call back. I have been told that they were just waiting for the lawsuit. The culture at the time was not to speak to anybody involved in a serious adverse event, but I did not know this.

Moving Forward

After a year I wrote a letter to the administration. I said that patients left their facilities all the time after something had gone wrong and asked why we were not supporting them. I offered to help them make the change. I received a letter back a couple of months later. It was very cold and written in legal terms. It made me so angry, I wanted to lash out and hurt them back. I remember thinking, "Now I know why patients sue!"

Then, finally, nearly 2 years after the event, Dr. van Pelt and I met. I was finally able to put a face to the man who was part of an event that had such an impact on my life. We had shared this extremely emotional event and I didn't even know what he looked like. By this time I had met a number of clinicians and I believed the system had failed us both. I wanted to change that. I remember telling him I wanted to start an organization, although at the time I had no idea what it would look like. MITSS—Medically Induced Trauma Support Services—had a brainstorming brunch in April of 2002, and Dr. van Pelt was one of the many invited guests. This was where we developed the mission of MITSS and ideas for how we would carry it out. Dr. van Pelt was one of the first board members of MITSS.

I was so naïve; I really thought that if I started this organization all the hospitals would send us the people who needed our support. I was so wrong. Three years to the day after my adverse event, I scheduled an appointment with the risk manager of the hospital. I had MITSS brochures and I was going there to see if she would give them to all her patients and family members. I left early, all ready for the meeting, and after I left she called the house canceling the appointment. So can you imagine the look on her face when I showed up? But we have become good friends, and she tells me now that they did not know what to do. They did not know what I wanted. They assumed I wanted something, but all I wanted was to be part of a solution. They could not comprehend that. It has taken years for me to build credibility with this hospital. What struck me was that if we are not acknowledging that these events happen, not doing disclosure or apology, then how can we get to the support piece? It has been a journey. I am now starting to see some progress, but it has been slow.

The institution finally made changes and promised to put our brochures throughout the hospital. But when I would go in, I would find our brochures on the shelves in the closets. Then Dr. van Pelt and I had our pictures on the front page of the *Wall Street Journal* and suddenly it was a different game. After this publication, I had the opportunity to meet with the hospital, and we were given office space at the hospital. Once I began to learn what the challenges were for the medical community we could look for solutions together, because sometimes they just didn't see them. They needed the patient's perspective. It has been a rewarding partnership. I wish people would take the opportunity to embrace their patients when things go wrong because amazing things can happen.

Conclusion

Seven years after the incident described in this chapter, Linda Kenney had her long-postponed ankle replacement surgery. While every effort was made to allay her and her family's fears before surgery, postoperatively she developed a surgical site infection that required rehospitalization and intravenous vancomycin antibiotics. After more years of acute issues and breakdown in the replaced ankle, Linda finally had the ankle replacement removed and a total ankle fusion in 2014. Her nonprofit organization, MITSS, has continued to grow during this time. It is now entirely consumer-led and is a leading source of information on supporting patients and healthcare professionals following medical harm.

Case Discussion

Linda Kenney relates the silence of the hospital following her near-death experience from medical error and the reluctance of the hospital to help her anesthesiologist reach out to her following her injury. Her story illustrates the ways in which the difficulties of communication magnify the psychological harm of an already traumatic event. The silence that Linda encountered was the traditional response to harm of many healthcare institutions, which included severing communication with injured patients and taking actions aimed at reducing legal liability rather than promoting healing. This response can leave both patients and healthcare professionals with a sense of abandonment, loss, and uncertainty (MITSS & Carr, 2009). Surveys have shown that the main things most patients and families want after medical harm are an apology, an explanation of what happened, and assurance that steps are being taken to bring meaning from their experience by preventing its recurrence. Anecdotal accounts also indicate that many healthcare providers remain troubled by adverse events throughout their careers (Conway, Federico, Stewart, & Campbell, 2011).

The movement toward more openness in dealing with adverse events in the United States began in the 1990s with Dr. Steven Kraman at the Lexington, Kentucky, Veterans Affairs hospital (Kraman & Hamm, 1999). It spread to the University of Michigan in 2001, where attorney Richard Boothman was a leader in developing a systematic program of disclosure, compensation, and patient safety improvement. Boothman also reported substantially reduced legal and insurance costs (Boothman, Imhoff, & Campbell, 2012). This model has been described as

emphasiz[ing] both honest communication with patients and families and a systems approach to errors. It promotes a principled institutional response to unanticipated clinical outcomes in which health care organizations (1) proactively identify adverse events, (2) distinguish between injuries caused by medical negligence and those arising from complications of disease or intrinsically high-risk medical care, (3) offer patients full disclosure and honest explanations, (4) encourage legal representation for patients and families, and (5) offer an apology with rapid and fair compensation when standards of care were not met. (Bell et al., 2012)

A similar philosophy emerged in Massachusetts in 2006 when the Harvard hospitals published a set of guiding principles based on the viewpoint of the harmed patient and stressing support of the patient (Massachusetts Coalition for the Prevention of Medical Errors, 2006). In 2012, a program based on these principles was piloted in six Massachusetts hospitals under the aegis of a consortium known as MACRMI, of which Linda Kenney's organization MITSS is a member. Though still far from universal, these principles have spread to many hospitals in the United States. One impetus for their spread has been the ineffectiveness of the legal system, which compensates only around 1% of medical error victims. Proponents of the full-disclosure model cite the perceived inhumanity of the court system toward both patient and provider and the impediment the traditional system poses to education and quality improvement because of lack of learning from mistakes. In most institutions that have adopted the full-disclosure model, adverse events are assessed using the "just culture" approach, which looks for the systemic cause of the event rather than penalizing individuals for mistakes (Bell et al., 2012; Conway et al., 2011).

Questions

1. How much of a problem do you believe the policy of not disclosing errors to patients might be? Can you envision circumstances in which this would create ongoing problems for patients and their families?

2. What adverse effects have you seen on clinicians who were involved in a medical error? What do you think could be done to alleviate these adverse effects?

3. Research some of the full-disclosure programs that have been developed and discuss their major components. What barriers do you see to provider disclosure following error? How do full-disclosure programs overcome the barriers to transparency that exist on both sides?

4. Much of this story is a lack of compassion in health care. Do you think there are forces that discourage compassion in day-to-day dealings with patients? If so, how do you think they could be overcome?

5. Which of the core competencies for health professions do you think are most relevant for this case? Why?

References

Bell, S. K., Smulowitz, P. B., Woodward, A. C., Mello, M. M., Duva, A. M., Boothman, R. C, & Sands, K. (2012). Disclosure, apology, and offer programs: Stakeholders' views of barriers to and strategies for broad implementation. *Milbank Quarterly, 90*(4), 682–705.

Boothman, R. C., Imhoff, S. J., & Campbell, D. A. Jr. (2012). Nurturing a culture of patient safety and achieving lower malpractice risk through disclosure: Lessons learned and future directions. *Frontiers of Health Services Management, 28*(3), 13–28.

Conway, J., Federico, F., Stewart, K., & Campbell, M. (2011). Respectful management of serious clinical adverse events (2nd ed.). IHI Innovation Series white paper. Cambridge, MA: Institute for Healthcare Improvement.

Kraman, S. S., & Hamm, G. (1999). Risk management: Extreme honesty may be the best policy. *Annals of Internal Medicine, 131*(12), 963–967.

Massachusetts Coalition for the Prevention of Medical Errors. (2006). When things go wrong: Responding to adverse events. A consensus statement of the Harvard Hospitals. Burlington, MA: Massachusetts Coalition for the Prevention of Medical Errors. Available at: http://www.macoalition.org/documents/respondingToAdverseEvents.pdf

Medically Induced Trauma Support Services [MITSS] & Carr, S. (2009). Disclosure and apology: What's missing? Advancing programs that support clinicians: A report based on an invitational forum held on March 13, 2009, sponsored by Medically Induced Trauma Support Services, Massachusetts Medical Society, CRICO/RMF, and ProMutual Group. Chestnut Hill, MA: MITSS.

Professionalism

Healthcare professionals must demonstrate a commitment to carrying out professional responsibilities and an adherence to ethical principles. Specific competencies within the Professionalism domain are to demonstrate:

- Compassion, integrity, and respect for others.
- Responsiveness to patient needs that supersedes self-interest.
- Respect for patient privacy and autonomy.
- Accountability to patients, society, and the profession.
- Sensitivity and responsiveness to a diverse patient population, including but not limited to diversity in gender, age, culture, race, religion, disabilities, and sexual orientation.
- A commitment to ethical principles pertaining to provision or withholding of care, confidentiality, informed consent, and business practices, including compliance with relevant laws, policies, and regulations.

Case 14, "The Big Picture: A Terminally Ill Patient in a Fragmented System," chronicles Fred Holliday's diagnosis and treatment of stage 4 cancer of the kidney. Fred and his wife Regina encountered poor health information systems, lack of access to Fred's medical chart, and a lack of communication among healthcare providers.

Linda Carswell writes about her husband Jerry Carswell in Case 15, "Without a Heart: The Legal Sequelae of an Unexplained Hospital Death." Jerry, a retired high school track coach, went to the hospital for a kidney stone. In the early hours of the morning when he was supposed to be discharged, Jerry was found deceased in his hospital bed. The family suspected medication error and narcotic overdose, and they became increasingly suspicious when the hospital was not forthcoming about the cause of death. Linda's account chronicles the lengthy legal battle that ensued.

Rita Hooper Washington's journey in the healthcare system is described in Case 16, "Small Steps: From Medication Adjustment to Permanent Disability." Mrs. Washington, who had been on warfarin therapy for many years, entered the hospital when she began bleeding after an increase in her warfarin dosage. Heart rate monitoring in the hospital indicated an irregular heartbeat, and doctors recommended a pacemaker, a decision that led to infection, disability, and a cascade of medical interventions over many years.

Case 17, "The Definition of Alive: The Story of an Equivocal Birth," is the tragic story of the birth and death of Paris Humphrey. Meg Humphrey tells the story about her pregnancy with Paris and the untoward events of her labor and delivery. Shortly after the birth, it was clear that the baby was lifeless, but doctors first prevaricated, and then disagreed as to whether the baby had died in utero or after birth. A protracted disagreement between the obstetrician and the neonatologist over who should sign the death certificate left the family in a legal and emotional limbo for over 2 years.

As in other sections of the book, we caution the reader that these cases are complex and include elements of other competencies as well. As you read the cases, it is helpful to think about the other competencies that are relevant. (Refer to the full list of competencies in the appendix.)

The Big Picture: A Terminally Ill Patient in a Fragmented System

The Story of Fred and Regina Holliday (United States)

Julie Johnson, Helen Haskell, and Paul Barach

Editors' Note

The following account is taken from an interview with Regina Holliday conducted on April 25, 2012. A painter and performing artist, Regina Holliday came to patient advocacy through the premature death of her husband, Fred Holliday, a university instructor in film studies. Regina has taken an unusual path in her campaign for patients' rights in her husband's memory. She speaks at medical conferences and meetings worldwide while producing paintings reflecting the themes of the meetings. Her 17-by-70-foot mural, "73 Cents," chronicling her husband's journey through a broken healthcare system, is one of several Holliday murals in public locations in Washington, D.C. (Eidolon Films, 2011). She also paints individuals' medical stories on the backs of business jackets. Regina has painted hundreds of jackets that are worn by patients, medical professionals, and others, who gather throughout the year in Washington and other venues as members of "The Walking Gallery" (Eidolon Films, 2013). She has been part of White House conferences, has spoken onstage alongside the U.S. Secretary of Health and Human Services, and has organized her own conference and advocacy group, Partnership with Patients (U.S. Department of Health and Human Services, 2010; Barr, 2013). She writes about her activities and those of others in a widely followed blog and Twitter account (Holliday, n.d.).

Prior to 2009, Regina and Fred led a very different life, renting a small apartment in Washington and working long hours to provide for their two young children. In her interview, Regina tells how their lives were upended after Fred was diagnosed with stage 4 kidney cancer at the age of 38.

LEARNING OBJECTIVES

After completing this case study, you will be able to:

1. Discuss the ways in which an integrated electronic medical record can contribute to improved care coordination.

2. Create strategies to engage patients and their families as partners in their care.

3. Assess the benefits of allowing patients real-time access to their medical records.

4. Appraise the role of social networks as a way to support patient communities and give healthcare providers feedback on their performance.

Scenic Painting

I grew up in Oklahoma and I went to Oklahoma State University where I met my husband, Fred. We met when we were both enrolled in a theater class called Scenic Painting. We were both procrastinators, and the night before a painting project was due we would both arrive at 10:00 p.m. and start painting. We would paint and we would fight. I don't know if you have pulled all-nighters with people on a regular basis, but all the filters come down. So we talked all night about religion and God and entertainment and Stephen King, because we were both huge Stephen King fans. And after an entire semester of throwing paintbrushes at each other and having huge arguments, we realized we had fallen in love in the best way you possibly can because you've seen it all already.

Well, time passed. We married and were living in Washington, D.C. We had two wonderful sons, Freddie and Isaac. By that time, my husband had a PhD in film studies, but we had a very limited income. Fred and I had six jobs between us. But even with six jobs we were living in a one-bedroom apartment and could not afford family health insurance. I was insured through my retail job in a toy store, but it didn't provide coverage for the rest of the family. Fred worked as an adjunct professor and a clerk and had no insurance. We only went for sick care, which meant that Fred didn't have a lot of continuity of records or information.

In the summer of 2008 our prayers were answered. Fred was hired in a 1-year full-time appointed position at American University. It was the job my husband had always wanted, and it carried full benefits, including health insurance.

"That's What the Doctor Said"

That fall Fred often complained of fatigue, but he thought, "Well, I'm working so hard at this new job; that's probably it." He was losing weight, but he had been getting fit and eating right, and we just thought he was doing a really good job with his diet. He went to the doctor and she said he had high blood pressure. We thought it was weird that he should be getting high blood pressure now, when he was so much thinner than he had been. But that was what the doctor said, so he was started on blood pressure medications.

In January the following year he started complaining of chest pain. He went to the emergency room, and they said he had broken a rib coughing. I was questioning it, but my husband said, "That's what the doctor said."

Then, in February, Fred started having lower back pain, to the point that he had to lie down all the time because it hurt to sit. He kept going back to the doctor, and she kept giving him pain medications. Then he developed another problem as a side effect of the pain medications, and she had to prescribe laxatives for that. By March he was on four types of painkillers, two types of muscle relaxants, four types of laxatives, and we still didn't know what was wrong.

On Friday March 13, my husband hurt so bad he was crying. I said, "Honey, they're not going to be able to get you in to the office. It's too late. It's 5:00 on a Friday afternoon. Let's go to the emergency room.

We can at least find out what's wrong with you." So I gathered up a bag of toys for the children and we went to the emergency room. We waited for about 3 hours until finally somebody came and said that they were backed up and we might as well go home. They gave Fred some more pain medications and said he should go see his doctor.

So the next week he went back to the doctor. This time I went with him because I thought, this has gone on too long. The doctor came into the examining room carrying a flip chart. She was looking down at the flip chart and she said, "So Mr. Holliday, do you think maybe you are depressed?" I said, "Of course he's depressed! He's in pain all the time, and you don't know what's wrong with him. We're worried. I think it's his kidneys."

And she said, "No, it's a protuberance of lumbar 5. Some people have this and don't need surgery, and some people do. So we'll just do some more x-rays and find out." I said, "No, we're going to do an MRI, because we need to find out what's wrong. And he is claustrophobic, so we want an open MRI and we want it this week." There was only one open MRI facility—in Olney, Maryland, a tiny town outside Washington, D.C.—that could see him that week. So Fred drove all the way out there and had the MRI. They gave it to him on a CD and he drove it all the way back into the city, handed it to her, and 4 days later she called us.

She said she wanted us to make an appointment with someone she knew who was an oncologist. I didn't even know what an oncologist was. I had to go online and find out. I said, "He just has a protuberance of lumbar 5. Why do we want to see a cancer doctor?"

She said, "We just want to make sure everything is all right."

Tumors and Growths

We went the next day to the oncologist. By this time Fred could hardly walk. They admitted him straight to the hospital for tests.

We waited 3 hours to get a room. Then after I got him all set up they said, "We're going to need all his pills." So I went home on the Metro system to get his pills and bring them back to them, so they could figure out what he was already on. I made sure Fred was comfortable and then I went home to take care of the kids. I thought I could do that. I didn't know you weren't supposed to leave a patient by himself.

A day later, on March 27, I'm at work selling toys. And my boss comes to me with the phone and he says, "Reggie, it's your husband." I answered the phone. Fred said, "Reggie, I'm so scared. The doctor was in my room and he says that I have tumors and growths in my abdomen, and he says that there is a 3-centimeter tumor in my kidney, and I don't know what's going on. Can you please get here as soon as possible?"

I left work and I got there in 30 minutes. I talked to my husband and calmed him down and said, "I'm going to find out what's going on." And I went to look for the doctor. But I found out that the doctor had left town in the last 30 minutes for a 4-day medical conference. He would not return phone calls or emails and there was no way to talk to him.

My husband's parents came into town, and we all sat in that room for 10- and 12-hour days, just waiting for someone to talk to us. On the fourth day, an on-call doctor came into the room. She walked right past us and went to look at the PCA pump. And we said, "What about his tests? What are the results?" She just looked at us. She said, "You mean nobody's talked to you? Nobody's told you?" We said, "No, we've been waiting for days. No one talks to us." And she said, "Oh! Well, it's spread. It's everywhere. It's in his bones and in his lungs."

So that night I went home and Googled what that meant. It meant my husband had stage 4 kidney cancer and he probably wasn't going to live more than a few months.

Little Miss A-Type Personality

When the doctor got back to town later that week he visited my husband during 7:30 a.m. rounds. I wasn't there yet because I was taking the kids to school. He said, "So I understand your wife has been asking questions about this case." My husband was a really good patient and didn't want to make waves, and the way he asked it frightened him. He said, "Yes, she's been asking questions." And the doctor said, "Well, if little Miss A-type personality has questions she needs to come to my office hours."

So I dressed in my church dress and I went at 9:00 in the morning to his office hours. He never closed the door in the 15 minutes I was there. He never stopped taking phone calls. He never turned the computer screen around so I could see what he was talking about. He didn't stop talking to the nurse about a parking lot problem where one employee kept parking in the wrong space, or that Mrs. Rose's chemotherapy suite wasn't ready for that afternoon and he needed it to be ready ASAP. When he talked to me, he used words I didn't understand and he spoke very rapidly.

I said, "Please, please, slow down, because I am writing everything down so I can research it later online." He said, "I don't like people who research online." I said, "Well, I don't have a background in medicine, so the only way I can understand you is to look these words up online." He said, "That's right. I'm the one with the medical degree." It felt horrible to be treated this way. It felt like Fred and I weren't part of the care team.

"Don't Worry About the List"

Fred's care at the hospital was terrible. His sheets were not changed for days. He was moved 20 times from bed to gurney even though he had a pathologic hip fracture. Once he could no longer walk to the bathroom I often had to change him myself and apply ointment I had brought from home. He was left for days with a dangerously distended bladder and never given a urinary catheter. They keep telling us they were trying to line up surgery for his kidney cancer, but it didn't happen.

Finally, after 3 weeks, I went down to the medical records department. I wanted the entire medical record. I wanted to see in writing what was wrong with my husband. And when I got down there they said it would be 73 cents per page and a 21-day wait. I said, "You mean it is going to cost hundreds of dollars to get my husband's medical record?" They said, "Well, yeah. That's just the way it is." "And I have to wait 21 days? He's upstairs right now!" They said, "That's just the system." So I went back to my husband's room.

About 9:00 a.m. the next day the doctor came in. He stood by the door, about 10 feet from the bed. I said, "We have the list!" We had a list of questions for him, things like: When are we going to get a palliative consult? When are we going to get a walker so he can try to walk again? And chemotherapy? And when are you going to give us surgery?

He said, "Don't worry about the list. We have decided we are sending you home on a PCA pump."

And that's when my husband began to cry. Because they were just sending him home to die. We had been there 3 weeks, we didn't know what was going on, and they were sending him home to die. And then the doctor left. My husband turned to me and said, "You go after them, Regina. You try to get me care."

It was a Saturday. I couldn't do anything that day or the next, but on Monday I fired the primary care doctor who never visited and I got my own primary care doctor to take my husband on. I called all the oncology practices to get a second opinion. I found a hospital willing to take him and I barred the oncologist from the room—everything to make sure we got better care.

Medical Facts

It took 3 more days, but we were transferred by ambulance to another facility. The first hospital was not helpful. When they sent us to the second hospital, they sent us with an out-of-date and incomplete medical record and transfer summary. It was 2 weeks old. So when Fred got to the new hospital, they could not provide care. All they could do was give him a bed. They said, "We can't even feed you, because you don't have dietary orders." The nurse said, "You can go down to the pizzeria and we'll pretend we didn't see you." That's how I fed my husband that night.

He was in excruciating pain because he didn't have any pain medication. I stayed at his side for the next 6 hours, trying to calm him down, until finally they cobbled together a medical record using a phone and a fax machine and were able to give him his pain medication. The next day, Fred's doctors came into the room, stood next to his bed and touched him and held his hand. Fred was so happy. Then they took me aside and said, "We want you to go back to the old hospital. We want you to get the entire medical record."

"Ha!" I said. "I tried that. They won't give it to me." They said, "Well, they will this time, because you're a courier."

I went back and they printed out the record in an hour and a half to give to the new doctors. I took it, and the new doctors read it for about an hour, and then they gave it back to me. They told me, "If you always have this medical record with you, your husband is going to get better care." So I read it in the next 3 hours. And I became so angry, because it was full of information, that if we could have only read it at the time we could have intervened and he wouldn't have suffered as much. There were also errors that we could have corrected if we had known. The words written in the record didn't reflect what actually happened.

When I saw his record, I thought, I may not have a medical degree, but I can paint about this. So I created a visual example, based on the nutrition facts label, of my husband's chart, everything that everybody should know about this man before they touched him. I even color-coded it, so you could see that these are the points of bone metastases and these are the points of soft tissue metastases; the fact that he's catheterized and incontinent. All these things just available at a glance, so you could give him appropriate care. And then I took this and I painted it on a wall. There was a delicatessen in my neighborhood and they had 5 × 6 feet of space and they said, "Yes, you can paint it there." It's right next to the menu in the delicatessen. And everybody, all our neighbors saw: this is what's going on.

Growing the Network

All this time I used Facebook as a way to keep people up-to-date on Fred's progress. I grew this huge network of people, and they are all still my friends today. They're all still supporting us. Then I got on Twitter because a toy store customer told me about a guy called e-Patient Dave, who had survived stage 4 kidney cancer.[1] I said, "I have to talk to e-Patient Dave! How do I talk to him?" They said, "You've got to get on Twitter."

So that night with the help of my 10-year-old autistic son, I got on Twitter and sent my first tweet. It said, "I want to find Christina Kraft or e-Patient Dave." The very next day e-Patient Dave found me, and by that night I was on the phone with e-Patient Dave's oncologist, a foremost authority on kidney cancer.

And that man was brave. He was willing to do "the talk." You know the talk? That sometimes it is too late. Sometimes you can be 38 years

---

[1] Dave deBronkart, or e-Patient Dave, is a kidney cancer survivor and a leader in the "e-patient," or participatory medicine, movement. The e-patient movement promotes active involvement of patients in their own health care and the use of electronic communication and social media to manage medical care and facilitate the exchange of information between patients. The "e" in e-Patient stands not only for "electronic," but also for "engaged," "empowered," "equipped," and "enabled." (Hoch & Ferguson, 2005; Mace, 2013).

old and the father of two young children and the day you get to the hospital, it's too late. That talk had never happened, ever, to any of us in the family. But this man from Twitter, he told me.

Through Twitter we met a lot of healthcare innovators from the e-health movement, Health 2.0.[2] I had a wonderful conversation with them, and they encouraged me to do something I had never thought of—blogging.

Conclusion

While these things were happening, Fred was moved to a hospice. Fred loved hospice. They took care of his pain. They didn't wake him up in the middle of the night. He was happy there. But after 3 weeks the discharge nurse came up to me and said, "Your husband's stable, so we need to send him home now."

I said, "But we have a one-bedroom apartment. How are we going to make that work?" They said, "Have you considered moving?" So we moved. In about a 24-hour time frame, with the help of 20 friends, we moved from a one-bedroom to a two-bedroom apartment that, thank God, was handicap accessible.

So I took my husband home. I only had four chucks (bed pads): I had one under him, one ready to go, one in the wash, and one in the dryer, to constantly keep him clean so he wouldn't get bedsores. I had bruises up and down my arms from trying to lift his body and care for him. We would only see a hospice nurse or a tech every other day. On the fourth day, the hospice nurse said to us, "You know, I think you should go back to hospice. This is not easy in your

---

[2] Health 2.0 is a movement that utilizes social media and other interactive capabilities of the Internet to promote an electronically networked approach to health care consisting of collaboration and data-sharing among patients, healthcare providers, and researchers (Eysenbach, 2008).

home." I said, "What?! You made us move! You made me uproot our whole family!"

"Well, that's how insurance works. You have to prove you're not able to do it and then you go back." I said, "No. This is not how it works. I swore to him, I promised him, that this would be the last move." And we stayed in our new apartment.

Then on the night of June 16, Fred called out, "Reggie, Reggie, my catheter blew!" I said, "Oh, it's okay, I'll clean it up." And I called the hospice nurse and she came in 2 hours. At 2:00 in the morning she was placing a new catheter and my husband said, "You are so good at that!" She said, "I was a VA (Veterans Affairs) nurse." And then she swept our floor. I said, "You don't have to sweep our floor." She said, "Just go be with your husband."

And then she left. And for the next 4 hours I just talked with my husband. It was just like Scenic Painting back at Oklahoma State. We talked about Stephen King and Jon Stewart and we talked about our kids and all these great things. And sometimes he didn't make sense. Sometimes he talked like he was talking to someone he knew when he was 6. But a lot of times it made sense; a lot of times it was my husband again.

Then at 6:30 he said, "Reggie, you look so tired. You should go to sleep." I slept for 1 hour, because his 7:30 medications were due. At 7:30 a.m. I got up and got his meds, but he wouldn't wake up. He moved his lips and managed to swallow, but he never talked again. Two hours later, he could hardly breathe. I ran for the children. I said, "Come on, kids. I think it's time." We gathered around the bed. And we said, "We love you, Daddy. We love you so much. But it's okay. It's okay to go. We will miss you, but it's okay."

And he stopped breathing. The hospice nurse came. She said, "Would you like to help clean the body?" So I held him, for the first time in weeks. He was warm. And I loved him so much.

Case Discussion

Regina Holliday felt compelled to action by her husband's experience in the hospital. Even before he entered hospice, she had, with Fred's blessing, met with healthcare activists, painted her first healthcare mural, and begun her healthcare advocacy blog. Five days after his death, she began painting the massive outdoor mural, "73 Cents," that chronicles in visual form the details of the story recounted above. Within 2 weeks she had begun combining the art, writing, social media, and public appearances that have been the hallmark of her activism. Regina has focused her advocacy largely on the poor health information systems that she and Fred encountered on their journey through the healthcare system: the lack of access to Fred's medical chart, the lack of communication between doctor's office and hospital, and between hospital and hospital. But the communication problems she captures in her art, writing, and speaking also raise the far larger issues of patient safety, healthcare quality, and access that were present in Fred's story.

Fred's case is an example of delayed diagnosis that, while it might not have changed the final outcome if addressed earlier, would definitely have provided him with better and more supportive care. The failure of the system to attend to the Hollidays' repeated questions and inquiries greatly contributed to the poor quality of care, as did Fred's admission to a hospital whose culture lacked both patient centeredness and attention to patient safety. Fred initially did not have health insurance, a fact that kept him from receiving routine medical care that might have detected his cancer earlier. When he did seek medical care, his cancer remained undiagnosed by a primary care physician who treated symptoms and did not look for underlying causes. Once diagnosed, he was in the care of an oncologist who was unavailable, arrogant, and dismissive. In the hospital, Fred was not given needed care such as a urinary catheter and even basic nursing care. Fred and his family were not only denied access to his medical record but also not given information about his condition that had a direct impact on decisions and quality of life.

Finally, the terminal nature of Fred's disease and end-of-life discussions were veiled in euphemisms and not discussed openly until mere weeks before his death, through an unplanned conversation with a doctor who had no association with Fred's care.

Questions

1. Review the instances of poor care coordination in Fred's case. Do you think that technology can provide the fix for these problems, or is the issue a lack of human teamwork and a system that does not accommodate the needs of patients and families?

2. What do you think are the factors that contribute to a delay in diagnosis in a case like Fred's, in which the patient is gradually but steadily declining? What in the working environment of the providers might have contributed to this failure to investigate the underlying cause of a patient's symptoms?

3. What changes do you think patient/family access to the complete medical record might bring to the medical system?

4. Do you see a role for the arts in health care? Do you think it is a worthwhile expenditure of scarce resources? Why or why not?

5. Regina Holliday emphasizes the importance of the Internet and social media such as Facebook and Twitter in the creation of communities of "e-patients" that she believes will change the practice of medicine. Look up "e-patients" and visit an online patient forum for patients with a serious medical condition. What effect do you think this medical model is having on medical practice?

6. Which of the core competencies for health professions are most relevant for this case? Why?

References

Barr, S. (2013). Activist ignites a movement for patients through art and story. *Kaiser Health News*, February 22.

Eidolon Films. (2011). 73 Cents: A grieving artist, a 50-foot wall, and a quest for patient rights. Available at: http://73centsfilm.com

Eidolon Films. (2013). The Walking Gallery of healthcare. Available at: https://vimeo.com/80009527

Eysenbach, G. (2008). Medicine 2.0: Social networking, collaboration, participation, apomediation, and openness. *Journal of Medical Internet Research, 10*(3), e22.

Hoch, D., & Ferguson, T. (2005). What I've learned from E-patients. *PLoS Med, 2*(8), e206.

Holliday, R. (n.d.). Regina Holliday's medical advocacy blog. Available at: http://reginaholliday.blogspot.com

Mace, S. (2013). What the "E" in E-patient really means. HealthLeaders Media, May 28. Available at: http://www.healthleadersmedia.com/page-1/TEC-292597/What-the-E-in-EPatient-Really-Means

U.S. Department of Health and Human Services. (2010). Press conference: Final rules to support meaningful use of electronic health records. Available at: http://www.youtube.com/watch?v=0jPSa-tfyKs

Without a Heart: The Legal Sequelae of an Unexplained Hospital Death

The Story of Jerry Carswell (United States)

Linda Carswell

Editors' Note

Linda Carswell and her husband Jerry lived for more than 25 years in Katy, Texas, a small town just outside Houston. The Carswells were both high school teachers; Linda taught English, and Jerry coached football and track. He was a beloved and highly success- ful coach who made it a priority to secure track scholarships for his runners, many of whom might not otherwise have been able to pay for a college education. In 1998, after winning the state track meet—an ultimate goal for Jerry—Jerry retired and took up an earlier career as a real estate agent. Jerry maintained close relationships with his former athletes, many of whom went on to become coaches themselves. Linda was proud of her husband's coaching and dedication to his students and the impact it had on their community.

At the age of 61, just 6 years after his retirement, Jerry went to the hospital for kidney pain. He was admitted for observation and soon began to improve. But early on the morning he was supposed to be discharged Jerry was found dead in his hospital bed, apparently after receiving a dose of narcotics. This is Linda's story of her husband's experi- ence in the hospital and of the medico-legal saga that followed his mysterious death and continues to this day. During the autopsy procedure, Jerry's heart was removed and retained by the hospital, an act that has been the cause of a highly publicized battle by his wife for its return.

LEARNING OBJECTIVES

After completing this case study, you will be able to:

1. Discuss the role of transparency of clinical information, in which patients and family members are given the full clinical story as well as access to the patient's complete medical records.

2. Discuss the implications of patients and family members being able to identify differences in training levels of health professionals at the bedside.

3. Debate the differences between forensic autopsy and clinical autopsy and the relative value of the information received from each.

4. Critique the role of the court system as a means of dealing with medical injury.

5. Discuss the role of the informed consent process for patient autopsy and retention of tissue samples at autopsy.

A Sudden Pain

One Monday morning in early 2004 my husband Jerry woke me and said his back was hurting. When the pain became severe we decided to go to the emergency room. At the emergency room, they treated him for the pain with several rounds of narcotics, including injections of morphine and Dilaudid. The emergency room doctor arrived and ordered a CT scan. When the CT scan results came back, the emergency room physician said that it looked as though Jerry was passing a kidney stone. Jerry was admitted to the medical-surgical unit for observation and pain management.

The hospital suggested a urologist, who visited us that afternoon. The urologist confirmed that there was a kidney stone but said the CT scan also had shown a small mass within the kidney. He wanted to do an additional test, with dye, to see the mass.

Jerry was given morphine and the painkiller Toradol (ketorolac) by intravenous injection every 4 hours through the night and into the following day. They also set up IV fluids to help wash out the kidney stone.

The next morning, Tuesday, Jerry was supposed to have a CT scan with dye to get a better look at the mass in his kidney. I went to school to prepare lesson plans in anticipation of being away from class. When I returned to the hospital, Jerry told me that they had not done the test because something was wrong. So I found a nurse, who said that Jerry's blood work had shown his serum creatinine level was rising. They did not want to perform the dye test until these kidney function test results looked better.

Jerry continued to receive Toradol throughout the day even though his pain was well controlled. I asked a nurse if this kind of high creatinine level was normal for a person with a kidney stone. She told me that it was probably caused by the Toradol and explained that nonsteroidal anti-inflammatory drugs like Toradol can cause the creatinine level to rise. She told me Jerry was getting too much Toradol.

This nurse was an RN—a registered nurse—but I did not realize this at the time. The nurses' badges did not designate whether they were an RN or a licensed vocational nurse (LVN). The attire was the same for all nurses, so I could not distinguish between them. The hospital's policy was to use RNs only as "resource" nurses. There were only two registered nurses on the floor, and they were not assigned to specific patients. The bedside nurses taking care of the patients were LVNs. So if an LVN needed to give a medication that she was not authorized to give, the LVN had to find a registered nurse who could administer the medication. I did not understand at the time that this was the policy.

When the doctor came to the room on Tuesday evening around 5:30, I mentioned Jerry's creatinine level and told him what the nurse had said. While the doctor was in the room his three pagers went off at various times, all while we were trying to have a conversation about Jerry. When I brought up the creatinine a second time, he told us he would discontinue the Toradol and restart the IV fluids to get the creatinine level down.

By 7:00 that night they still had not started the IV fluids. When the night shift nurse came in, she told me there had been no order placed for this request. At my insistence, she called the doctor, and later she started the IV and discontinued the Toradol. At that time, Jerry's pain medication was changed to a Lortab tablet every 4 hours because his pain level was now only about 2 on a scale of 1–10.

On Wednesday morning I dropped by the hospital and then I went on to school. Around noon Jerry called and asked me to come back to the hospital. He said they were trying to explain something to him but he could not understand because the medication was making him feel confused. So I arranged for a substitute teacher for the afternoon and returned to the hospital.

I stayed with Jerry throughout the evening. About 7:15 that evening the bedside nurse (an LVN) came in with medication. Jerry told her he was not going to take it because it was making him feel odd and his pain level was minimal. The LVN told him that he needed to maintain his pain relief regimen, but Jerry refused the Lortab. He told her that if he needed the medication he would let her know. I left the hospital about 8:00 that evening, as our son Jordan had come to visit Jerry. They watched basketball and talked politics until around 9:00 p.m., when Jordan left the hospital.

Jerry was set to go home the next morning. We were just waiting for results of the morning blood test to confirm that his creatinine level had come down so that he could be discharged. Because the CT scan with dye had not been done, Jerry was scheduled for an MRI after discharge because the hospital did not offer open MRI services. His pain was minimal and manageable with Lortab, so the doctor had told Jerry he could leave the hospital to get the MRI and follow up after the doctor's office had received the images.

Your Husband Is Dead

The following morning, Thursday, January 22, the phone rang at 5:50 a.m. I thought it must be Jerry because when he was away from home he would often call early in the morning to say good morning. The person on the phone told me that my husband had had an emergency and that I needed to come to the hospital immediately. When I asked what had happened, she said there had been an emergency and a urologist was in with him now. She asked how long it would take me to get to the hospital. I said about 5 minutes. I was terrified. She had given me no information about my husband's "emergency." I assumed because a urologist was with him that he was passing the kidney stone and that something had happened related to the kidney stone.

I dashed to the hospital and ran up to the second floor where Jerry's room was. As I entered the waiting area I saw our son. At that moment my heart stopped. A nurse I had never seen before came walking toward me as I started down the hall to Jerry's room; she took Jordan and me into an empty patient room. The nurse looked at me and said, "Your husband is dead." I was absolutely stunned. This could not be true. I kept repeating, "No! No!"

A young woman who was standing with the nurse told us that pain medication had been given to Jerry sometime in the early morning hours. She was crying as she told us this. I learned later that she was the new on-call attending physician for the urology group. She had only recently finished her residency. She had never seen Jerry before but had been called to the hospital when the staff discovered that Jerry was dead.

The nurse repeated to me several times, "Your husband died peacefully in his sleep. You can take comfort in that." At that point, I ran out of that room and into Jerry's room, and he did look asleep, except that there were tubes inserted into his mouth and I saw a catheter hanging on his bed. The room was nice and neat, and Jerry was lying on his back with his hands on his chest. It all looked surreal.

My shock was so complete that I tried to wake Jerry—tried shaking him—finally collapsing in screams and sobs. The same nurse stood in the doorway and said again, "He looks like he is just sleeping, doesn't he? Doesn't he look peaceful?"

The young doctor who had told us about Jerry's death was gone. I asked again and again what had happened, but we could not get anyone to answer any specific questions. When I asked about the tubing and the catheter, the nurse said they had called a code and that a full resuscitation with intubation was standard procedure. A nurse came into the room some time later and asked if we wanted the tubes removed. I said, "No, don't change anything." I did not want anything changed because I did not know what had happened.

During that morning I questioned nurses and the administrator who had come in to talk to us. I kept receiving the same news—that Jerry had died peacefully in his sleep. The administrator asked us about funeral arrangements, and a nurse brought in a release form. I asked about the county medical examiner. Had he been called? When would someone come to begin the investigation? The nurse told me that the medical examiner's office was "not interested in investigating" Jerry's death. I was stunned. I asked, "What did you tell them about the cause of his death?"

She replied, "Renal failure."

Again, I was shocked. I knew for certain that his death was not caused by renal failure. Just a few hours ago, Jerry had been in minimal pain, talking, laughing, and watching basketball. There had never been any mention of renal failure. We later learned that the Harris County medical examiner's office had no record of a call from the hospital about Jerry's death. A representative from that office gave a sworn affidavit attesting to "no record of a call concerning Jerry Carswell" received from the hospital.

I told the hospital administrator that I wanted an autopsy. Jerry was supposed to come home, he had no other health problems, he was taking no other medications, and he had been active. The nurse told me that the urologist had already ordered an autopsy. I asked how that worked. Did they do them here or somewhere else? The nurse said they would do the autopsy at a hospital in downtown Houston. I told her that I did not want the hospital where Jerry had died to perform the autopsy, because I wanted an independent autopsy. The nurse replied that an autopsy could cost up to $10,000. At this point I did not care how much it might cost; I just wanted it to be complete so I could find out what had happened. Jordan and I talked this over—we wanted an autopsy that would tell us why Jerry had died.

A nurse brought me the document to request the autopsy. She assured me that the autopsy conducted by the hospital would be "just like" an autopsy I would get from an independent patholo-gist. There was a place to mark if I wanted a partial autopsy or anything specific. I wrote on the paper, "Complete Autopsy," and signed it.

At one point the hospital administrator came into the room and announced that it was "time for us to go home." I told her I wanted to be there when the funeral home transported Jerry's body out of the hospital. I again stated that I did not want anything removed from Jerry's body, and I specifically requested that the urine from the catheter bag go to the autopsy. Later, around noon, the admin-istrator came back in and told us the funeral home was on their way to transport Jerry's body for autopsy. She literally placed her hand on my back and pushed me toward the door of the room. We all then left the hospital and went home. Later, I learned that the funeral home did not arrive at the hospital until more than an hour later.

There are no adequate words to describe what I felt like leaving the hospital, the reality of the cold air when I got outside, of what had just happened inside that building. Jerry was gone. I could not absorb that fact, or that I had just signed for an autopsy when I had never before had any occasion even to think about an autopsy, or the fact that no one at the hospital would tell us anything specific about how Jerry died. There I was, going back home alone—this surely was some terrible nightmare.

Looking for Answers

When I went home, I called friends, and they called friends, and by the next day the *Houston Chronicle* published a story in the sports section about the loss of this man whom everyone in the area knew. There was an outpouring of response from coaches in the area and from the students Jerry had coached. His death was a great loss to many people.

While we were mourning his loss, Jerry's body was being transferred to the pathology lab at the hospital in Houston. The autopsy was done there. But it turned out that this hospital was a sister hospital to the one where Jerry had died. It was not the independent autopsy we thought we were getting.

We later found that there are two distinct kinds of autopsy procedures. Clinical autopsies, the kind usually done in hospitals, do not include the same investigative procedures that a forensic autopsy does. Even though a large dose of narcotics had been administered to Jerry prior to his death, Jerry's autopsy did not include toxicology screening that would have been done by the medical examiner or by an independent pathologist in what is called a forensic autopsy. Jerry's autopsy was done by a pathologist who testified that he had never done a toxicology screen in an autopsy, not once in his 20+ years of working for that hospital pathology group. The pathologist did not test the urine that remained in the body. The urine bag that I had seen in the hospital room disappeared. A hospital pathologist said the bag was not with the body when it arrived in the lab.

Shortly after Jerry was buried, I went to the hospital and got his records. When I read the report from the emergency room doctor who had been called to the code, it said that Jerry had been found lying across the bottom of the bed as if he had been trying to get up. The urologist's report said the same thing. This was in direct conflict with what I had been told at the hospital, that he had "died peacefully" in his sleep.

That is the point at which I decided I needed more information. The attending urologist from the hospital helped us get the autopsy report, but he never answered my questions about why there were two conflicting stories. The hospital did not return my calls.

When we received the death certificate, there was no cause of death listed. We still, even now, do not have an official cause of death. The death certificate listed three conditions present prior to death. These had to do with an irritation in the lining of Jerry's stomach and in the pyloric area, both of which we believe were probably side effects of the Toradol and not underlying conditions; Jerry had no indication of any kind of medical distress other than the kidney stone until we came to the hospital. Ironically, the autopsy report showed no kidney stone on the right side where Jerry's pain had been. It noted a small stone on the other side still in the kidney. It also noted the small mass and said it "appears confined to the kidney."

After seeing Jerry's medical records, I talked with a friend who encouraged me to contact an attorney to see if we could find out what had caused Jerry's sudden and unexpected death. We then entered a long and difficult legal process that I wish we had not had to do. In that process we discovered a number of issues that were very disturbing.

One key issue was that the amount of the medication Toradol that Jerry had been given was far in excess of the strict limits recommended for this drug. This explained why the drug had such an adverse effect on his kidneys. Another was that the LVN who was administering the Toradol was not allowed by hospital policy to administer this class of drug and did not have sufficient training in the purpose of the drug or its possible side effects, which include adverse effects on the kidneys. Because the RNs were floaters and were not assigned to specific patients, there was no real monitoring or oversight of the bedside LVN nurses.

We also discovered that just before midnight on the night Jerry died, the same LVN had written details in Jerry's chart about giving pain medication to a knee surgery patient. She had detailed the angle the knee was positioned in and things like that. By the time we saw the records, this information had been lined out. The correction was initialed and dated January 22, the morning of Jerry's death, indicating to us that Jerry's LVN had not noticed her mistake during the night that Jerry died. Personnel records showed that this LVN had taken many extra shifts that week— more than twice the hours of any other nurse. I am not sure what mental state she was in the night of Jerry's death, but she definitely placed the wrong information in Jerry's record. As part of the correction done after Jerry's death, she reported that she had administered Lortab to Jerry about 1:00 a.m. We wondered if she could have given him the Lortab and the surgery patient's medication, too.

Jerry's records reflect a call to the on-call urologist saying that Jerry had been in level 9–10 pain since 1:00 a.m. At 3:15 a.m., according to the medication record, a nurse—it is unclear which nurse—administered a bolus does of 75 mg of Demerol and 25 mg of Phenergan. In trial, a laboratory technician stated she encountered two nurses coming out of Jerry's room with a syringe at 5:00 a.m. There is no record of a 5:00 a.m. medication administration, however. When the lab tech entered the room around 5:15 a.m. to draw blood, she found Jerry's lifeless body.

It was a year before we sought legal recourse, but in the end we felt we had no choice. The legal process was slow and stalled repeatedly for various reasons, including changes in hospital ownership. The hospital was uncooperative, and the judge sanctioned them for spoliation and destruction of evidence. The hospital mounted an unsuccessful challenge against both the sanctions and our requests for evidence. Then the hospital where the autopsy had been done filed for bankruptcy. All told, it took us 5 and a half years to get into a courtroom. When we finally got there, the hospital administrator and nurses denied under oath that they had ever spoken to Jordan and me about the funeral home or the autopsy. This was proven not true by funeral home documents and by the testimony of other people who had been present that morning.

The jury vote fell two votes short of the number required for a negligence verdict in Texas. Several jurors later stated to my attorney that because there was no official cause of death, they felt there were too many unanswered questions to make a determination, even though they felt that the hospital had caused Jerry's unexpected death. The jury voted in our favor on the post-mortem fraud, finding that the statements hospital personnel made to me had led me to believe the autopsy would be "complete" and would be an investigation into the cause of Jerry's death. In a unanimous vote, the jury added punitive damages as a punishment for what they considered the hospital's egregious misconduct.

Conclusion

One of the most shocking things to come out of the lawsuit occurred during the pathologist's deposition. He stated that he had removed Jerry's "whole heart" and retained it in his lab. The pathologist did not request permission or inform me that he had retained Jerry's heart and stored it in an unmarked plastic bucket in the pathology lab. We had buried Jerry without his heart, a disturbing and painful realization that haunts us still.

I became convinced that Texas needed a state-promulgated consent form for autopsy so that families could be informed about their rights concerning autopsies. In addition to Jerry's heart being removed without our knowledge, Jerry's death met three of the six conditions that Texas law specifies as requiring a death investigation or forensic autopsy. I went to my state representative and asked him to sponsor a bill that would require hospitals to use an "informed consent" for autopsy, a document that would inform families of their legal rights. The Jerry Carswell Memorial Act passed the Texas legislature in 2011, and now every medical institution in the state must use this form when they ask for permission to do an autopsy. The form lists the conditions under which state law says there must be a death investigation and states that the patient's family has the right to request an independent pathologist to attend or perform the autopsy (**Figure 15-1**).

Case Discussion

Jerry Carswell entered the hospital for flank pain that was thought to be due to a kidney stone. His hospital stay was prolonged by abnormal laboratory values apparently brought on by incorrect dosing of the nonsteroidal anti-inflammatory drug ketorolac. After his pain had diminished and he was preparing for discharge, Jerry died suddenly from an apparent narcotic overdose. Although the hospital was not forthcoming about the circumstances surrounding his death, Jerry's wife thinks he may have been given drugs intended for another patient and that nurse fatigue and lack of oversight may have contributed to the error.

Much of the dispute in the case revolved around the topic of autopsy. Jerry's autopsy, performed at the request of his wife, was a clinical autopsy, which did not include the toxicology screening that might have revealed the narcotic overdose his family considered the most likely cause of death. Clinical autopsies are done in a hospital and require the permission of the family. A forensic autopsy of the type Linda Carswell believed had been performed is a more detailed death investigation, usually performed by medical examiners or coroners under circumstances in which investigation into cause of death is required by law (Sanchez, 2013). A century ago, clinical autopsies were considered essential to medical learning, and a 20% autopsy rate was required for accreditation by The Joint Commission until 1970. Since that requirement was dropped, the autopsy rate in American hospitals has plummeted, and autopsies are rare unless mandated by law (Burton, 2014).

TEXAS DEPARTMENT OF STATE HEALTH SERVICES

POSTMORTEM EXAMINATION OR AUTOPSY CONSENT FORM

This form is prescribed under Article 49.34 of the Code of Criminal Procedure. Please see the reverse side for further information regarding the law and the completion of this form.

NAME OF DECEDENT:	DATE OF DEATH:
NAME AND TITLE OF PHYSICIAN PERFORMING PROCEDURE:	TEXAS LICENSE NUMBER:
NAME OF FACILITY AND DEPARTMENT WHERE THE PROCEDURE WILL BE PERFORMED:	

The physician may be required to remove and retain organs, fluids, prosthetic devices, or tissue for purposes of comprehensive evaluation or accurate determination of a cause of death.

....

Please indicate which, if any, restrictions or special limitations you would like to make on the procedure:

☐ None. Permission is granted.

☐ Permission is granted for an autopsy with the following limitations and conditions (specify):

____ Exam is restricted to brain and spinal cord   ____ Exam is restricted to the chest and abdomen only

____ Exam is restricted to the chest cavity   ____ Exam is restricted to the abdominal cavity

____ Other: (Specify) _____

....

I authorize the release of the remains to the funeral services provider or person listed below after examination.

Name of Funeral Service Provider or Person:	Telephone Number:

_____   _____

Authorizing Person's Signature   Date

_____

Authorizing Person's Printed Name and Relationship to Decedent

_____   _____

Witness's Signature   Date

_____

Witness's Printed Name

Warning: It is a felony to falsify information on a Vital Statistics application, record or report. The penalty for knowingly making a false statement on this form or for signing a form which contains a false statement is 2 to 10 years imprisonment and a fine of up to $10,000. (Health and Safety Code §195.003)

Figure 15-1. Postmortem Examination or Autopsy Consent Form

Reproduced from Texas Department of State Health Services "Postmortem Examination or Autopsy Consent Form" VS-200, 04/2012.

TEXAS DEPARTMENT OF STATE HEALTH SERVICES

POSTMORTEM EXAMINATION OR AUTOPSY CONSENT FORM

This form <u>MUST</u> be completed by the person authorized to give consent to a postmortem examination or autopsy before such procedure can be conducted [CCP Art. 49.32].

This form IS NOT required if an autopsy is ordered by a Justice of the Peace or Medical Examiners as part of an death inquest or ordered by the Texas Department of Criminal Justices under Texas Government Code §501.055 [CCP Art. 49.31].

Persons Authorized To Consent to Postmortem Examination or Autopsy

Consent for a postmortem examination or autopsy may be given by any following persons, who are reasonably available, in the order of priority listed:

- the spouse of the decedent;
- the person acting as guardian of the person of the decedent at the time of death or the executor or administrator of the decedent's estate;
- the adult children of the decedent;
- the parents of the decedent; and
- the adult siblings of the decedent.

If there is more than one person of the same relation entitled to give consent to a postmortem examination or autopsy, consent may be given by a member of the same relationship unless another person of the same relationship files an objection with the physician, medical examiner, justice of the peace, or county judge. If an objection is filed, the consent may be given only by a majority of the persons of the same relationship of the class who are reasonably available. An example of this would be multiple surviving adult children.

A person may not give consent if, at the time of the decedent's death, a person granted higher priority as listed above is reasonably available to give consent or to file an objection to a postmortem examination or autopsy.

Anatomical Gift by Decedent Prior To Death

An anatomical gift of a donor's body or part may be made during the life of the donor for the purpose of transplantation, therapy, research, or education by

- the donor,
  - o if the donor is an adult; or
  - o if the donor is a minor and is:
    - emancipated; or
    - authorized under state law to apply for a driver's license because the donor is at least 16 years of age and:
      - circumstances allow the donation to be actualized prior to 18 years of age; and
      - an organ procurement organization obtains signed written consent from the minor's parent, guardian, or custodian;
- an agent of the donor, unless the medical power of attorney or other record prohibits the agent from making an anatomical gift; a parent of the donor, if the donor is an unemancipated minor; or
- the donor's guardian.

Anatomical Gift of Decedent's Remains by Someone Other Than the Decedent

Unless the decedent has refused to make an anatomical gift in writing prior to death, an anatomical gift of a decedent's body or part for the purpose of transplantation, therapy, research, or education

Figure 15-1. *(Continued)*

may be made by any member of the following classes of persons who is reasonably available, in the order of priority listed:

- an agent of the decedent at the time of death who could have made an anatomical gift under Section 692A.004(2) immediately before the decedent's death;
- the spouse of the decedent;
- adult children of the decedent;
- parents of the decedent;
- adult siblings of the decedent;
- adult grandchildren of the decedent;
- grandparents of the decedent;
- an adult who exhibited special care and concern for the decedent;
- the persons who were acting as the guardians of the person of the decedent at the time of death;
- the hospital administrator; and
- any other person having the authority to dispose of the decedent's body.

If there is more than one member of a class listed above entitled to make an anatomical gift, an anatomical gift may be made by a member of the class unless that member or a person to may be receiving the anatomical gift and knows of an objection by another member of the class. If an objection is known, the gift may be made only by a majority of the members of the class who are reasonably available.

A person may not make an anatomical gift if, at the time of the decedent's death, a person in a class higher than them is reasonably available to make or to object to the making of an anatomical gift.

Death Inquest by Medical Examiners

Some deaths may require a medical examiner to conduct an investigation or inquest and cause of death certification which may include an autopsy. [CCP Art. 49.25 §6]. These include:

- A body was found and the cause and circumstances of the death are unknown.
- The death is believed to be an unnatural death from a cause other than a legal execution (accident, suicide, or homicide).
- The death occurred in prison or in jail.
- The death occurred within 24 hours of admission to a Hospital
- The death occurred without medical attendance.
- The physician is unable to certify the cause of death.
- The deceased is under six (6) years of age.

Nonaffiliated Physicians

Before signing this form, a representative of the hospital or other institution where the death occurred is required to inform a person authorized to consent to a postmortem examination or autopsy that they may request that a physician who is not affiliated with the hospital or other institution where the death occurred to perform the postmortem examination or autopsy at another hospital or institution.

A person authorized to consent to a postmortem examination or autopsy may also have a physician that is not affiliated with the hospital or institution where the death occurred review the postmortem examination or autopsy conducted by a physician affiliated with the hospital or other institution where the deceased person died.

A person requesting a nonaffiliated physician to perform or review a postmortem examination or autopsy is responsible for any additional costs incurred as a result of the nonaffiliated physician's performance or review of the examination or autopsy.

Figure 15-1. *(Continued)*

The Carswells' belief that the hospital was not honest with them about Jerry's death caused them much distress and led them to turn to litigation to find answers. At the trial, the jury found the hospital guilty of fraud for withholding information from the family about the completeness of the autopsy that would be performed and the independence of the laboratory that would perform it. The hospital's response to Linda was described as "a material, false misrepresentation with at least reckless disregard for the truth" in the ruling by a three-judge panel of the Court of Appeals for the First District of Texas (2013). In a supplemental opinion issued in April 2014 by this same court, the court refers to the "wrongful cover-up of its negligent acts . . . that [the hospital] was found to have conducted in this case" (Court Of Appeals For The First District Of Texas, 2014).

The longest-standing issue in the case has been the removal and retention of Jerry Carswell's heart, which the family says was done without their knowledge (Allen, 2011, 2012, 2013). Although members of the public are generally unaware of it, organ and tissue retention is permitted and not uncommon in autopsy. In the United Kingdom, the Alder Hey scandal led to the revelation that organs from thousands of children had been retained for educational purposes. This in turn led to national reforms requiring transparency in consent for autopsy and organ retention and return (BBC News Health, 2001; McDermott, 2003). The United States, however, has no standard national policy. A sample form published by the College of American Pathologists (2009) suggests that families should be explicitly informed of their rights to set restrictions on clinical autopsies, including restrictions on organ retention, but not all states require this. One of Linda Carswell's achievements in her husband's name has been the creation of an autopsy consent form for Texas.

Nearly 10 years after Jerry's death, the hospital continued to fight the return of the heart tissue, saying it could be important evidence in the ongoing legal battle. In August 2013, the appeals court determined it should be returned to the widow. Upon testing of the heart, it showed no human DNA (Allen, 2014). The reasons for this are not clear, but as of this writing the heart remains unburied.

Questions

1. What do you think Jerry Carswell's nurses and doctors could have done to protect against the adverse outcome that occurred?

2. What steps do you think the hospital should have taken to avoid the suspicions and antagonisms that immediately arose between this family and the hospital?

3. Consider the legal process in this lengthy case from both the hospital's and the family's point of view. Is this the best way to handle this situation?

4. Should more autopsies be mandated? Read some of the literature on autopsy findings and discuss whether you think a high autopsy rate is a good idea.

5. Look up the differences between forensic and clinical autopsies. Should toxicology screening be required in hospital autopsies?

6. Which of the core competencies for health professions are most relevant for this case? Why?

References

Allen, M. (2011, December 15). Why can't Linda Carswell get her husband's heart back? ProPublica. Available at: http://www.propublica.org/article/why-cant-linda-carswell-get-her-husbands-heart-back.

Allen, M. (2012, July 12). Cardiac arrest: Hospital refuses to give widow her husband's heart. ProPublica. Available at: http://www.propublica.org/article/cardiac-arrest-hospital-refuses-to-give-widow-her-husbands-heart.

Allen, M. (2013, August 30). One step closer to getting her husband's heart back. ProPublica. Available at: http://www.propublica.org/article/one-step-closer-to-getting-her-husbands-heart-back.

Allen, M. (2014, February 21). Hidden in a heart, a discovery 'beyond belief.' ProPublica. Available at: http://www.propublica.org/article/hidden-in-a-heart-a-discovery-beyond-belief.

BBC News Health. (2001, January 29). Organ scandal background. Available at: http://news.bbc.co.uk/2/hi/1136723.stm.

Burton, E. C. (2014). Autopsy rate and physician attitudes toward autopsy. Medscape Reference. Available at: http://emedicine.medscape.com /article/1705948-overview#a1.

College of American Pathologists. (2009). Sample autopsy consent and authorization form. Available at: http://www.cap.org/apps/docs /committees/autopsy/sample_autopsy_consent_form.pdf.

Court of Appeals for the First District of Texas. (2013). Opinion issued August 29 in The Court of Appeals for the First District of Texas, In Re Christus Health Gulf Coast (as an Entity, D/B/A Christus St. Catherine Hospital, and formerly D/B/A Christus St. Joseph Hospital), No. 01-12-00667-CV.

Court of Appeals for the First District of Texas. (2014). Opinion issued April 1 in The Court of Appeals for the First District of Texas, In Re Christus Health Gulf Coast (as an Entity, D/B/A Christus St. Catherine Hospital, and formerly D/B/A Christus St. Joseph Hospital), No. 01-12-00667-CV.

McDermott, M. B. (2003). Obtaining consent for autopsy. *BMJ*, *327*(4), 804–806.

Sanchez, H. (2013). Autopsy request process. Medscape Reference. Available at: http://emedicine.medscape.com/article/1730552-overview# aw2aab6b2.

Small Steps: From Medication Adjustment to Permanent Disability

The Story of Rita Hooper Washington (United States)

Julie Johnson, Helen Haskell, and Paul Barach

Editors' Notes

Rita Hooper Washington is a retiree living in Houston, Texas. She worked for 36 years as a claims coordinator for a large insurance company. In 2008, at the age of 58, Rita was admitted to the hospital for an adverse event related to her warfarin therapy. While in the hospital, heart rate monitoring suggested an irregular heartbeat, which prompted physicians to implant a pacemaker. The pacemaker incision site became infected, leading to lifelong disability for Mrs. Washington. The following account of the chain of events that led to her disability is taken from interviews with the editors in 2012 and 2013.

LEARNING OBJECTIVES

After completing this case study, you will be able to:

1. Describe the cascade effect in health care and how it can lead to inappropriate care.
2. Discuss the narrow risk margins of high-risk drugs such as warfarin and how patients can be better prepared to deal with these dangers.
3. Discuss elements of a patient-centered approach to informed consent.
4. Outline strategies for encouraging patients to be informed consumers.

Background

In 2008 I had been taking a medication called warfarin for about 15 years because I have a history of blood clots. They don't really know what caused them, but I have had eight bouts of blood clots. The first blood clot was in my lung (a pulmonary embolism) and the others were in my legs (deep vein thrombosis, or DVT). I had a venous filter installed in 2005 (an intravenous filter to help prevent clots propagating to the lungs from the legs).

I was told I would need to take warfarin the rest of my life and that it would keep my blood thin and would keep clots from forming. I get my blood INR[1] checked regularly to be sure I have the right level of warfarin and that my blood is not too thin.

In March of 2008 my doctor increased my warfarin level from 6 mg to 9 mg a day. A few days later, on March 15, I left my job early, about 12:30 in the afternoon, because I had profuse vaginal bleeding. This was on a Saturday. I went home immediately and called my doctor's office because I was planning on staying home. However, my doctor's nurse explained to me that when you are bleeding after taking warfarin you cannot take the risk of sitting at home, so I went immediately to the emergency room. While I was in the emergency room they decided that they were going to admit me to the hospital to find out why I was bleeding.

Good News and Bad News

My cardiologist came into my hospital room the next day and told me he was going to run some tests to try to figure out what the problem was. They put a portable monitor on me to measure my heartbeat. They had already discontinued my warfarin to try to get my INR levels back to normal. They gave me medicine to try to

---

[1] INR stands for International Normalized Ratio. The INR is a method of standardizing the results of tests of the clotting tendency of blood. The INR takes into account variations in the tissue factor used in the reagent when measuring prothrombin time.

control the bleeding, but it didn't work. During this whole time I continued to have vaginal bleeding.

On the third day in the hospital my blood count was so low that they decided I would need a blood transfusion. But when they gave me the transfusion that night I had an adverse reaction. As soon as the blood started going in I began to feel very cold. My breathing got short, and I started shaking uncontrollably. I heard the nurse run out and call a code STAT. Then I passed out. The next thing I knew, I woke up and I was no longer on the general medical ward. I had been moved to a room on the cardiac floor.

At noon the next day, the cardiologist came in to see me. He explained that he had some good and bad news for me. I asked him what the good news was. He said that they thought my INR was going down a little bit, but the bad news was that during the night the monitor had shown that I had an irregular heartbeat, and that it was a dangerous rhythm that could lead to sudden death. He said that I was going to need a pacemaker. I asked him what the pacemaker had to do with my bleeding, and he could not answer that question. He said that our biggest concern was to implant the pacemaker.[2]

I had no reason to not believe the cardiologist. However, no one brought me test results to show that I had irregular heartbeats during the night. I just went by what my doctor said.

The doctor kept saying that it was urgent that I sign the consent to get a pacemaker. However, I was more concerned at this point about the bleeding. I had not come into the hospital for a pacemaker. In fact, I had been in the hospital for chest pains just 2 months before, in January. They had run a stress test, and they had told me there was nothing wrong with my heart.

[2] Editors' note: Mrs. Washington was recorded as having a Mobitz Type II second-degree atrioventricular block, a serious condition that can lead to complete heart block, although it can also sometimes be mimicked by other conditions. The treatment for a Mobitz Type II second-degree atrioventricular block is an implanted pacemaker (Wogan, Lowenstein, & Gordon, 1993).

When I got out of the hospital in January I had also been seen by a doctor for sleep apnea. After I was told I had to have the pacemaker, my sleep apnea specialist came to see me in the hospital. He told me he did not think I needed a pacemaker, and that he was going to discuss this with my cardiologist. But the next day my cardiologist was out of town. His partner at the cardiology clinic came in and told me they had spoken with my sleep specialist and they really thought I needed to get the pacemaker. At that point, it was as if every doctor who came in was pressuring me to sign the consent for the pacemaker. I did not know what to do.

My sister was with me. She wanted me to get a second and third opinion, and I explained to her that I had seen other doctors. However, I did not relay to her that all these doctors were in practice together. My pastor and his wife were there with me, and they, too, questioned the doctor about the pacemaker.

I did not have the pacemaker implanted until 10 days after I was admitted to the hospital. One reason was that I did not want to make this decision while my regular cardiologist was out of town. This caused a delay, because I waited for him to get back. But when he came back he supported the other cardiologists in saying that I should have the pacemaker implanted.

I agreed to go ahead with the procedure, but I felt pressured. The procedure was canceled once because I was still bleeding, and they had to get my blood clotting under control. Finally I was taken down to the catheterization lab. My regular cardiologist did the procedure. I was given a sedative and I don't remember much, but I did not feel that I had any major problems. But the next morning when the doctors made their rounds and removed the gauze and tape they noticed that the area did not look right. My doctor had an infection control doctor come in. He believed it was a hematoma, or blood under the skin, and they immediately started me on an antibiotic in case it was infected.

Everyone's Body Is Different

Before I left the hospital, I was still having problems with my INR levels. When they discharged me I was back on warfarin and also still taking the antibiotic. I went home and took the medication they had prescribed. However, at night, for 2 nights in a row, the wound bled where they had placed the pacemaker. I was concerned about this. I called my cardiologist and he told me it was normal, that it was just drainage. At the end of the week I was still having problems, so I called back and asked if there was any possible way that I could come in and they could check it. So I went in and they told me it was normal. He said everyone's body is different. He told me I just needed to keep cleaning the area.

The wound was purple because of the bleeding. It was swollen and painful. The cardiologist kept telling me this was normal. His direct words were, "Your body is trying to adjust to having a mechanism in your chest." This did not make it better.

I went back to the infection control doctor for the first time on Friday, April 11, 2008, about 2 weeks after the pacemaker had been implanted. The wound was beginning to come open. Immediately, the infection control doctor said that the area was probably infected and sent me to the hospital. I had surgery that day to clean out the pocket where my pacemaker was implanted. On Sunday the doctor sent a nurse in with a form stating that I was going to have to undergo another revision of the pacemaker pocket. The doctor did not come to examine me or explain the need for the surgery and sent a message through the nurse that he would explain it to me on Monday before the operation. So on Monday I had more surgery on the area where the pacemaker was implanted. He did talk to me before the surgery, but it was never clear to me why I needed two surgeries.

During my next check with my cardiologist the nurse privately told me that by now I should have been healed from my first surgery back in March. A friend gave me the name of a cardiologist in the main medical center downtown. I went to see that doctor on May 14.

This doctor was an electrophysiologist. He looked at the pacemaker area and told me it was infected and that he would see me in surgery. The doctor explained that whenever you have any kind of device in your body, especially if it is up around your heart, there is no such thing as trying to repair it. It has to be taken out or it can do more harm to your body with more infections.

The next day my pacemaker was removed due to the infection. I stayed overnight to have intravenous antibiotics in the hospital and then took 10 more days of antibiotics at home. I never learned what kind of bacteria caused the infection.

After the pacemaker was removed my new cardiologist stated that we were going to wait 6 weeks and that at that point we would see if I needed another pacemaker. But then he expanded his practice and I started seeing him in the same office as my original cardiologist. After 6 weeks, when I asked him about putting in a new pacemaker, he saw my original cardiologist passing by in the hall. He went out and they had a long conversation in Spanish that I could not understand. He came back in and told me that we would not talk about a pacemaker again. That made me think that maybe I never really needed a pacemaker.

Two weeks later I had to go back in for a follow-up check-up. I still had some drainage, but it was not as bad as it was from my first surgery. (This was my fourth surgery at this point.) I asked what the next procedure would be after this because I had severe pain in the area where my pacemaker had been and radiating up my left shoulder and arm. The doctor said they would set me up to see a pain management doctor.

So the following week I started seeing a pain management doctor in the downtown medical center. He gave me numerous pain medications, but nothing really could ease the pain. I underwent physical therapy for about 3 months, and I continued to follow up with the pain management doctor.

During all this time I had taken leave from my job. Then when I wanted to go back to my job they did not have a position for me, so I had the choice of either taking a leave of absence or retiring. When I called my manager she just suggested that if at all possible I should retire. So that is what I ended up doing.

I continued with my physical therapy. Finally my pain management doctor told me that if the pain persisted I might need to go see an orthopedic specialist. So I did go see an orthopedic specialist, and he too prescribed more physical therapy and more pain medication. Finally the orthopedic specialist explained to me that I could start getting shots. I did not know what type of shots he was talking about, but it was a shot in the shoulder area. I had several shots, and each one would work for about a week.

After my fourth surgery the pain management doctor told me that due to the number of surgeries that I had had there was a possibility that I could have a frozen shoulder. I asked him what could be done to correct it. He said that over a period of time if the medication and the physical therapy did not work that we might consider surgery. I did not like this answer because this would be my fifth surgery. But I finally did have the surgery, and it did not help.

I have been without a pacemaker since May 15, 2008. I have never had anyone tell me whether or not I needed a pacemaker to begin with. They have never addressed this issue.

Conclusion

After all these procedures and events I lost faith in doctors and their clinics. While in physical therapy, when I was in pain I was told that I just needed to increase my exercises to improve my pain. I had to explain to them that I knew my own pain level, that I knew what my body was supposed to feel like, and that this was not normal. The pain in my shoulder has never gone away, and this has been since 2008. The level of pain that I deal with is at a level of 8 out of 10. I do exercises on my shoulder at home and nothing has ever seemed to get better.

I would say the most important thing for a patient is to have a good patient–doctor relationship. If you go to see a doctor who can only go in to talk to you for less than 5 minutes, then you need to get another doctor. Because you are paying that doctor and they are taking care of your health, you should demand that this doctor spend more than 5 minutes with you. I recommend that patients ask questions and ask their doctors to talk in terms that patients understand.

Before I had the pacemaker implanted, I tried to set up a friendly relationship with my doctor. But at some point, I just felt there was a lack of communication. He said I needed a pacemaker because the study showed that I had an irregular heartbeat. But I have had an irregular heartbeat since 1984, and he knew this because he had performed a stress test on me in January 2008. He did not tell me what had happened; he did not show me any proof that I needed a pacemaker.

If I had to do this all over again with the things I know now, I would have demanded that my doctor sit down and go over details with me to show me how my condition had deteriorated. Then I would have needed the doctor to address the main concern of why I came to the hospital. That was for my bleeding, which was never really addressed, other than by taking me off the warfarin.

Case Discussion

Rita Hooper Washington went into the hospital for an adverse event related to her medication therapy. While in the hospital, monitoring suggested an irregular heartbeat, which prompted physicians to implant a pacemaker. The pacemaker incision site became infected, leading to lifelong disability and several subsequent surgeries for Mrs. Washington. This is called the *cascade effect*, defined by Mold and Stein (1986) as "an initiating factor (or factors) followed by a series of events that seem to be a direct result of the previous events that proceeds with increasing momentum, so that the further it progresses, the more difficult it is to stop." Cascade events can be appropriate—Mold and Stein point out that the cascade of events that occur following the arrival of a patient to the emergency department without a pulse and respirations can trigger a series of life-saving steps. However, cascade effects can be triggered inappropriately, such as by an incomplete and/or inaccurate history and physical, error or misinterpretation of lab values, or underestimation of the risks of treatment. Although each small step in the sequence can seem logical, when put together they expose the patient to a preponderance of risk over benefit.

One of Mrs. Washington's big concerns is doctor–patient communication. She is particularly concerned that doctors often do not speak in plain language that patients can understand. Mrs. Washington is also concerned that doctors do not always take the time to listen to patients' concerns and to make sure that they are understood. Involving patients in clinical decisions has been recommended as a strategy for avoiding cascade effects (Deyo, 2002).

This caution applies to other healthcare professionals as well. Analyses of sentinel events suggest that poor communication among healthcare professionals is a leading cause of poor care (Cassin & Barach, 2012). Communication failure was given as the root cause of three-fourths of adverse events and close calls reported to the U.S. Department of Veterans Affairs' National Center for Patient Safety (Salas, Baker, King, & Battles, 2006; Dunn et al., 2007). The Joint Commission also cites poor communication as the most frequent cause of events in its sentinel events database and notes that "effective communication, which is timely, accurate, complete, unambiguous, and understood by the recipient, reduces errors and results in improved patient safety" (The Joint Commission, 2007; Leonard, Graham, & Bonacum, 2004).

Questions

1. What do you think went wrong with the informed consent process when Rita Washington was told she needed a pacemaker?

2. Track the cascade of events that Rita Washington experienced. Was there a point at which it logically could have been stopped? Should it have been?

3. What do you think healthcare professionals can do to improve communication with patients?

4. What can healthcare professionals do to maximize their time with patients and ensure that communication is effective?

5. Given that these are complex topics, what are basic precautions that can be taken to try to avoid medication error and infection?

6. Which of the core competencies for health professions are most relevant for this case? Why?

References

Cassin, B. R., & Barach, P. R. (2012). Making sense of root cause analysis investigations of surgery-related adverse events. *Surgical Clinics of North America, 92*(1), 101–115.

Deyo, R. A. (2002). Cascade effects of medical technology. *Annual Review of Public Health, 23*, 23–44.

Dunn, E., Mills, P., Neily, J., Crittenden, M. D., Carmack, A. L., & Bagian, J. P. (2007). Medical team training: Applying crew resource management in the Veterans Health Administration. *Joint Commission Journal on Quality and Patient Safety, 33*(6), 317–325.

Leonard M., Graham S., & Bonacum, D. (2004). The human factor: The critical importance of effective teamwork and communication in providing safe care. *Quality and Safety in Health Care, 13*(Suppl 1), i85–i90.

Mold, J. W., & Stein, H. F. (1986). The cascade effect in the clinical care of patients. *New England Journal of Medicine, 314*(8), 512–514.

Salas, E., Baker, D., King, H., & Battles, J. (2006). Special section commentary: Opportunities and challenges for human factors and ergonomics in enhancing patient safety. *Human Factors, 48*(1), 1–4.

The Joint Commission. (2007). National patient safety goals. Available at: http://www.jointcommission.org/standards_information/npsgs.aspx.

Wogan, J. M., Lowenstein, S.R., & Gordon, G. S. (1993). Second-degree atrioventricular block: Mobitz Type II. *Journal of Emergency Medicine, 11*(1), 47–54.

The Definition of Alive: The Story of an Equivocal Birth

The Story of Paris Humphrey (United States)

Meg Humphrey

Editors' Note

Meg Humphrey and her husband eagerly anticipated the birth of their third child, Paris. Meg was fit and healthy, her pregnancy was uneventful, and standard labor and delivery of a healthy infant was expected. Because Paris, like Meg's previous babies, appeared to be an unusually large baby, the obstetrician scheduled induction of labor at 39 weeks of gestation. But when Meg went for a routine check-up shortly before the scheduled induction, she was running a low-grade fever and experiencing irregular contractions, nausea, and diarrhea. The doctor admitted her to the hospital. Meg's labor course was remarkable for a brief episode of high fever and instances of decelerations on the fetal monitor. After the baby's heartbeat appeared to stabilize, Meg's labor progressed, and she had a normal vaginal delivery. Shortly after the birth, it became obvious that the baby was dead. The doctors disagreed about whether the baby had died in utero or after the birth.

LEARNING OBJECTIVES

After completing this case study, you will be able to:

1. List strategies to enable a prompt and accurate response to signs that a patient or fetus may not be doing well.

2. Discuss ways that healthcare professionals should respond when they see other professionals make a mistake.

3. Consider how healthcare professionals can assist each other when an adverse event happens.

4. Explore ways to deliver bad news to patients and families.

5. Propose strategies to deal with the uncertainty surrounding adverse outcomes and their aftermath.

No Sign of Life

I became pregnant with my third child in 2003. My baby, Paris, was delivered on September 3, 2003, at 39 weeks. I had assumed I could do this easily. The day before Paris was born my doctor's appointment was uneventful. Everything seemed fine. The baby was moving. The nurse connected me to a machine, and I heard the baby's heartbeat loud and clear. But I felt sort of sick to my stomach and I had a low-grade fever. The doctor said I was ready to have the baby and that she would induce me the following day.

I checked into the hospital around 5:00 that afternoon. I kept telling the nurses that I was not feeling well, that my stomach was upset. During the evening my fever rose to 102 degrees Fahrenheit. The nurses gave me Tylenol and I felt better. I had been having cramps throughout the day and I started to go into natural labor. My previous pregnancies had been induced, so I had no understanding of what it felt like to go into natural labor. I thought that maybe my not feeling well was part of that process. The nurses monitored my contractions and decided to give me Pitocin to hasten my labor.

The nurses were concerned that my water had not broken, and after about 30 minutes they used an instrument to break it. About an hour later, there was a moment of panic when they said the baby's heartbeat had stopped. All of a sudden the nurses came running into the room and jerked me up, placed me on all fours, and jiggled my belly trying to get her heartbeat back. It came right back, and they said it must have been faulty equipment. They reported this to the doctor, and the doctor ordered an intrauterine fetal monitor. They placed a little tiny screw into the baby's forehead. They said that way they would not confuse my heartbeat with her heartbeat. But after a while the heartbeat disappeared again. They said, "It must be a faulty screw." They placed another one and then they heard a heartbeat again.

At that point, they decided to let my labor progress. My friends were there, my husband was there, my in-laws were there, my mother was coming, and our children were aware that the baby was coming. Everything was very normal. The doctor arrived, and about 30 minutes later I delivered a beautiful 8-pound, 14-ounce baby. She was huge. The doctor held her up and said, "It's a girl!" They placed her in the warming bed right next to me.

There was no sign of life. The baby didn't move and I didn't hear her cry. I knew something was wrong. I immediately asked, "Why isn't she crying?"

Their response was, "She's fine; she just needs to be startled."

We had a video camera there to record her birth, so there is a video of the baby being delivered by the physician. The video shows a nurse placing a mask over the baby, and it shows the baby looking very bruised and purple. She never cried or moved. The nurse was very young and very distraught. In the video you can hear me saying over and over, "Why isn't she crying?" Once we knew that something was wrong the camera was shut off.

The doctor then ordered that the baby be taken out of the room. About 20 minutes later, a neonatal doctor came in and said, "Your baby is not doing well; we don't know why."

I asked, "Is she okay?"

She said, "We have hooked her up to machines."

I asked, "Is she breathing?"

She said, "The machines are helping her breathe."

I asked, "Is she moving?"

She said, "She is not moving."

I was not sure at this point what the definition of "alive" was. What I had just seen was a baby that did not look alive, but then again, maybe she just needed to be startled. The neonatal doctor left and came back again. I asked the same questions, and she gave me the exact same answers.

My husband asked again, "Is the baby alive?" What I didn't know was that my husband was watching the nurses and they were just standing there. No one was doing anything, because the baby was clearly dead. He knew the answer to the question, but they weren't comfortable telling us because there were no answers. My husband was waiting for the neonatal doctor to tell us our baby was dead.

We asked, "If we turned off the machines, then what would we have?" The doctors' response was, "Then your baby would be dead."

So we asked them to turn off the machines. There was no life.

Finding out What Happened, Who Said What and When

After that it rapidly became about who said what and what had happened. I sat in the hospital and dealt with the social workers. It was very awkward and uncomfortable. They brought the baby to me, and I remember them asking me if I wanted to hold her. I thought that was bizarre. I had my family and the staff and nurses in the room with me and they were waiting to see my reaction. I remember holding her and being so uncomfortable with all the eyes on me. I held her for a few minutes and then gave her back to the nurse.

During this time the doctor was trying to prove her case to me, showing me the baby's heartbeat on the monitor strip and telling me she had done everything she could. She kept asking me to look at the printouts. Of course I had no idea what I was looking at. She said the equipment was not used scientifically, that it was just a monitoring system. I wasn't quite sure what this meant. The doctor said the monitors were not a diagnostic tool, and that it was not her fault if they weren't used properly or if they didn't work.

I was moved into another wing of the hospital, and we started planning our daughter's funeral. Then my blood cultures came back. They showed that I had a staph infection, that the baby had a staph infection, and that her levels were much higher than my levels. This was the first clue. How does a baby in a uterus get levels of staph that are higher than the mother's?

I really didn't care much about any of that at the time. I just cared about getting out of the hospital, but they made me stay several more days to take IV antibiotics. I went home with IV medication, and a nurse came to my home to change the IVs for several weeks.

As they were planning to take the baby to another hospital for the autopsy, they came to me and said, "Before we take your baby to perform the autopsy, would you like to hold her?" I was alone then, and that was the only time that I spent with her. This was a very special time for me. Even though she was cold and stiff it was a very special moment for me. I am glad that they asked me. They also took pictures and did a hand mold and gave me all the clothes that she was wearing. They placed me in contact with a support group. They did helpful things on that end. It was very different from the actual delivery when so many mistakes were made.

We had so much to adjust to at that time that we didn't ask many questions. But after our daughter's funeral, the questions began. I started questioning everything that had happened and wanted to know if things could have been different. Our pediatrician helped me set up an interview with the pathologist who had done the blood cultures. The pediatrician came with me, and they allowed me to record the interview. The pathologist went through every page of the report. They said the infection was not MRSA; it was treatable staph. No one could explain why Paris's levels were higher than mine, why she was so much sicker than I was. I never was very sick. They tested my kidneys and did some other tests and found nothing wrong with me, but Paris's body was completely destroyed.

The confusing part was that the hospital where I delivered claimed that I delivered a live baby with an APGAR of 1, but the autopsy done at the children's hospital said that the baby was deceased for more than 6 hours before birth. This would have put the death around the beginning of my time on all fours, when they first lost the heartbeat. That would mean that later on they must have been picking up my heartbeat and thinking it was the baby's, because at this point the baby was already dead. On the fetal monitor strips, my heartbeat and the baby's were both recorded as being around 120 after that time, so it was certainly possible.

Because the hospital said she had been born alive, Paris was issued a social security number and a birth certificate and treated as a live birth. But once you have a live birth, in order to close out a person's life, you need a death certificate. I could not get a death certificate because no physician would sign it. The physician who delivered the baby stated the baby was born alive; she refused to sign the death certificate because this would mean that the baby died with her, and she said that she gave the neonatologist a live baby. The neonatologist said she would not sign the death certificate because she was given a dead baby. This caused a lot of problems and heartache for us. Not only did we have to make arrangements for our dead child, we had to fight to prove that she was dead.

We could not get any help with this. Finally, after 2 years, the doctor who had delivered the baby signed the death certificate. She waited to sign until the 2-year statute of limitations—the period of time during which you are allowed to sue in the state of Texas—had elapsed. She shouldn't have worried. We had decided not to sue the hospital or the doctors, but I have always been troubled by the death of my daughter and how the care providers behaved.

Conclusion

The autopsy found that I had a staph infection that was transmitted to the baby before birth, but they never found a source of staph infection in my body. It was in the baby's body. Her levels were ridiculously high. Mine were only moderately high. My blood cultures came back showing that I had a staph infection, but there was no boil or cut, no obvious natural way for infection to have entered my body.

I don't know if the doctors knew Paris was dead when she was born. That is the confusion. The obstetrician never told me why she thought the baby was alive. In fact, I did not ask that immediate question. When I tried to follow up with her in the hospital I was not allowed to talk to her. My care had been transferred to an infectious disease doctor instead. I did demand to see the original doctor at my 6-month check-up, and I asked her questions then. She was very remorseful and said it had never happened before. She said, "I have a hard time even seeing patients right now. Every time a patient comes in and says they don't feel well I want to rush and take the baby out." This helped me, to know that it mattered to her. Her mistake was that she didn't do a cesarean section the minute there was trouble. She allowed me to continue labor and then placed the blame on the equipment.

I was bothered by the way the nurses talked to me when Paris was born. I was so vulnerable; I was in stirrups. I did not understand what was going on, and I was looking to them for direction. The nurse was young and had probably never suffered a loss and clearly never had any training in dealing with a dead baby or with grieving parents. She kept saying the phrase "fetal demise," which is a very harsh phrase to hear when you don't know what it means. My daughter's name was Paris. She had clothes ready to go home, and she had an entire nursery set up at home. I needed someone to use her name and look me in the eye and talk on my terms. I needed them to recognize her as a human being and not a number or a last name.

We still have so many unanswered questions. I do believe Paris was born dead. In my mind she was delivered dead. What was going on during the delivery I don't quite understand, but I believe that she suffered during that time. It will never stop bothering me. But I feel that at some point we have to make sense of it as best we can, put it away, and continue on with our other children and family.

Case Discussion

Meg Humphrey's story is an account of poor communication and conflicting interpretations surrounding her daughter's birth. The autopsy in the case of baby Paris resolved some of these questions and raised others. It indicated that the cause of death was a fulminating staph infection, apparently contracted shortly before birth. But the baby had extensive damage to her brain and other organs that usually takes many days, and even weeks, to develop. The pathologists believed the damage had occurred earlier in the pregnancy, possibly as the result of a prior infection. This suggests that the baby's prognosis was in question even before birth.

Although it is not clear how the baby contracted the infection that led to her death, it is abundantly clear that her birth and delivery involved a series of failures in communication and judgment on many levels. First, there remains the question of why, in the face of signs of maternal infection and fetal decelerations, the baby's distress was not recognized. Could members of the team have been more vigilant, and if they had intervened earlier might the baby have been saved? Second, when the baby was delivered dead but was declared a live birth by the obstetrician, other members of the team appear to have been at a loss as to how to react and what to say to the family. Were the team members afraid to speak up and say the obvious when the obstetrician told the parents that the baby was alive?

The family's grief and confusion were compounded by insensitive behavior on the part of the clinicians involved. The family saw the obstetrician as focused on self-exoneration rather than helping them cope with their unexpected loss. The delivery room nurses did not know how to handle a situation of loss and used technical language that the parents found confusing and unfeeling. Although a team specialized in bereavement offered Mrs. Humphrey considerable solace in the latter part of her hospital stay, the obstetrician did not make herself available to the family in the days following the birth. Finally, a protracted disagreement between the obstetrician and the neonatologist over who should sign the death certificate left the family in a legal and emotional limbo for over 2 years.

Questions

1. The obstetric team seems to have confused the mother's and baby's heartbeat on the fetal monitor. What assumptions might have contributed to this confusion? Research the topic of cognitive bias and discuss biases that might prevent a timely response to medical problems in situations like this.

2. The baby's heartbeat was repeatedly lost during Meg Humphrey's delivery. Her care team attributed the anomalous readings to faulty equipment. In her communication with the parents after the birth, the doctor also blamed the insensitivity of the equipment for failure to recognize the baby's deterioration. Is this a reasonable excuse? What techniques can be employed to be sure you are getting correct readings from equipment? Explore the field of human factors and ways that devices can mislead clinicians.

3. Health care often involves trying to make sense of unclear information. What strategies can be employed to help deal with uncertainty in medicine? How and when should this ambiguity be communicated to patients and families?

4. What policies or procedures might have offered guidance to the members of the healthcare team when the obstetrician declared the baby to be alive when she clearly was not alive? Were the staff too fearful to speak up? Explore the importance of psychological safety as a measure of a culture of safety. Would you say the culture at this hospital was a safety culture or a fear-driven culture?

5. Meg Humphrey says that her delivery room nurses did not know how to deal with her loss or know how to talk to a newly bereaved mother. What should the nurses have done? How can this behavior be taught to healthcare professionals?

6. What is your interpretation of the standoff between the two doctors who refused to sign baby Paris's death certificate? Do you believe this violates professional and moral ethics? If so, in what way?

7. Which of the core competencies for health professions are most relevant for this case? Why?

Recommended Reading

Conway, J., Federico, F., Stewart, K., & Campbell, M. J. (2011). *Respectful management of serious clinical adverse events* (2nd ed.). IHI Innovation Series white paper. Cambridge, MA: Institute for Healthcare Improvement.

Emereuwaonu, I. (2012). Fetal heart rate misrepresented by maternal heart rate: A case of signal ambiguity. *American Journal of Clinical Medicine, 9*(1), 52–57.

Gold, K. J. (2007). Navigating care after a baby dies: A systematic review of parent experiences with health providers. *Journal of Perinatology, 27*(4), 230–237.

Gosbee, J. (2002). Human factors engineering and patient safety. *Quality & Safety in Health Care, 11*, 352–354.

Leonard, M., Graham, S., & Bonacum, D. (2004). The human factor: the critical importance of effective teamwork and communication in providing safe care. *Quality & Safety in Health Care, 13*(Suppl 1), i85–i90.

Systems–Based Practice

Healthcare professionals must be able to demonstrate an awareness of and responsiveness to the larger context and system of health care, as well as the ability to call effectively on other resources in the system to provide optimal health care. Specific competencies within the Systems-Based Practice domain are to:

- Work effectively in various healthcare delivery settings and systems relevant to their clinical specialties.
- Coordinate patient care within the healthcare system relevant to one's clinical specialty.
- Incorporate considerations of cost awareness and risk-benefit analysis in patient- and/or population-based care.
- Advocate for quality patient care and optimal patient care systems.
- Participate in identifying system errors and implementing potential systems solutions.
- Perform administrative and practice management responsibilities commensurate with one's role, abilities, and qualifications.

Glenda Rogers writes about her daughter, Robin Rogers, in Case 18, "Not for IV Use: The Story of an Enteral Tubing Misconnection." Robin was admitted to a hospital in Kansas for early induction of labor when she was 35 weeks pregnant. Robin and her unborn daughter, Addison, died from the effects of an enteral feeding solution that had been infused into Robin's intravenous central line, the result of a tubing misconnection.

Case 19, "Death Despite Known Drug Allergy," is about a woman in Australia who died after taking an antibiotic prescribed to treat an ear infection. Zoya (not her real name) had a history of allergic reactions, and her medical records clearly documented her drug sensitivities. The prescribing error was not detected when Zoya's doctor wrote the prescription due to the use of a hybrid medical record system whereby the prescription was written on paper and the progress notes were entered electronically after the patient had left the examination room. The error was also not detected when the medication was dispensed by the pharmacy. Zoya died from anaphylaxis after taking one tablet.

Case 20 is written by Lisa Morrise and Kirsten Morrise and tells the story of Kirsten, who was born with a genetic condition called Pierre Robin sequence. "The Trial Meant for You: The Lifelong Medical Journey of a Child with a Complex Congenital Condition" recounts the Morrises' experiences and lessons from a lifetime of medical intervention, beginning with the events surrounding Kirsten's birth when failure to recognize her condition led to a series of preventable errors.

As in other sections of the book, we caution the reader that these cases are complex and include elements of other competencies as well. As you read the cases, it is helpful to think about the other competencies that are relevant. (Refer to the full list of competencies in the appendix.)

Not for IV Use: The Story of an Enteral Tubing Misconnection

The Story of Robin and Addison Lowe (United States)

Glenda Rodgers

Editors' Note

Glenda Rodgers is a veteran nurse with more than 25 years' experience in obstetric nursing and several years' experience working in implementation of electronic medical records. Glenda's daughter Robin Lowe was a nursing technician in a family practitioner's office. Robin wanted to be a nurse like her mother and was planning to go to nursing school.

At the time of the events described in this case, Robin was married and had a 3-year-old son. She was pregnant with her second child, a daughter whom she and her husband Jeremy had named Addison. On a summer morning in her eighth month of pregnancy, Robin went to the emergency room with severe nausea and abdominal pain, a condition that had been an issue throughout the pregnancy. She was admitted to the hospital for early induction of labor. By the end of the day Robin and her unborn daughter were dead from the effects of an enteral feeding solution that had been infused into Robin's intravenous central line, the result of a tubing misconnection. The following is Glenda Rodgers's account of her daughter's medical history, the events surrounding Robin's hospitalization, and the untimely deaths of Robin and Addison Lowe.

LEARNING OBJECTIVES

After completing this case study, you will be able to:

1. Explore the scientific field of human factors and how errors like tubing misconnections can be prevented.

2. Discuss the complexity of having two patients to treat, a mother and her fetus.

3. Describe suitable actions by healthcare staff following the discovery of an error.

4. Discuss engineered forcing functions and how they can be used to make medical devices safer.

Background

On July 18, 2006, my daughter Robin was admitted to the hospital. She was 24 years old, and she was 35 weeks pregnant. She was admitted for intractable pain, vomiting, and dehydration.

It wasn't the first time Robin had been admitted to the hospital. She had had episodes with similar symptoms from the time she was 11 or 12 years old. She would have intense abdominal pain and would start vomiting. She would vomit 30 times a day. She would get dehydrated, of course, and so we would have to admit her to the hospital. The first summer it seemed like she was in the hospital every other week. The doctors finally decided it was an autoimmune syndrome that they had seen mostly in teenaged girls, and they just grow out of it. We tried allergy-type treatments, which never seemed to work, and in the end they decided that the only way they could treat it was symptomatically.

When she would get sick she would be admitted to the hospital and given intravenous fluids, and she would essentially take nothing by mouth until her stomach settled down and she could tolerate food again. She didn't get sick because of the nausea; she got sick from the pain and responded to narcotics. They would give her prednisone because of the allergy reaction, and they would hydrate her. And that's what we did for several years. As she got older, the episodes got fewer and farther between. By the time she graduated from high school, she was only getting sick two or three times a year. She got married and moved away and started working for a family practice doctor who prescribed medication she could take on a regular basis. She did well on the medication, and she seemed to have things under control.

Then she got pregnant. Her medication was not compatible with pregnancy, so she had to go off it. But she did fine, even after that, until she got to 28 weeks pregnant. And then, maybe because of the size of the uterus and the body changes, she became sick again. By the time she was 32 weeks pregnant, Robin had lost about 60 pounds. They decided to put in a central venous catheter, a catheter placed in a large vein in her chest. This let her take lipids and total parenteral nutrition (TPN), so she received most of her nutrition intravenously. She continued to work. She would come home and hook up her IVs; they would run all night, and she would go back to work the next day. Whenever she did start to get sick, she would go to the emergency room. They would give her some narcotics, which was an issue for some of the nurses because they didn't think she should get narcotics while pregnant.

During the last 3 weeks of her first pregnancy she basically quit eating and lived on ice chips, because anything she ate she threw up. They delivered her early at about 37 weeks. Jerick, my grandson, weighed 6 pounds, 4 ounces. Her weight loss hadn't bothered him at all. He did fine.

"It'll Be Different This Time"

Robin talked about wanting to have a little girl, and I kept discouraging her. I said, "Robin, you remember how sick you were. Do you really want to go through that again?"

Then Jerick came up to me one day and he had on a tee shirt that said, "I'm the big brother." I looked at Robin and said, "Oh, honey, really?" She said, "Yeah, Mom, but don't worry. It'll be different this time." I said, "Okay." I was thrilled, of course, to have another grand-child, but I certainly didn't want to see her in as much pain as before.

And again, she did well until she was 26 or 27 weeks along and then she became sick. Robin's younger sister was getting married in June, and toward the end of May, Robin's doctor, who was also the doctor that she worked for, wanted to put in a peripheral intravenous cen-tral catheter (PICC) running from an IV site in her arm to the large blood vessel above the heart to restart the intravenous nutrition. Robin didn't want to have a PICC line because she didn't want it to show in the wedding pictures. So she made him wait until the wedding was over, and about the middle of June they put in the PICC line. She began to infuse the TPN at night and continued to work during the day, just as she had done during her first pregnancy. She had probably lost 40 pounds by that time.

They did a lot of ultrasounds to make sure that the baby was grow-ing. We found out it was going to be a girl. She was just thrilled. She had her boy and now she was going to have her girl, and this would be the end of it. She wouldn't have to go through this again.

Jerick turned 3 on July 15 and we went to celebrate his birthday. Robin was very sick. I talked her into letting me take Jerick home with me so that they wouldn't have to worry about childcare if she had to go to the hospital. So Jerick came home with me.

On the morning of July 18 Robin called and said she had gone to the hospital. She was 35 weeks pregnant, and the doctor who was taking care of her wanted her induced. He talked to the pediatrician, and the pediatrician agreed. He said, "You know, she's 35 weeks. It's probably just as safe for the baby to be on the outside as it is on the inside, as sick as she is now."

Robin was excited. She said, "Mom, pack some extra clothes, because you're going to stay and we're going to have the baby." We were both excited. I started driving to her hospital, but when I was about halfway there she called and she was crying. She said the OB doctor, the obstetrician who was supposed to induce her, said he would not induce her before she had completed 37 weeks due to the risk to the premature baby.

He told Robin he didn't care how many times she got sick, that she would have to stay in the hospital until she was ready to be induced at 37 weeks as that was best for the baby. Well, that meant 2 more weeks in the hospital, without Jerick. She didn't have any extra time left to take off from work, and it was just devastating for her to find out that they weren't going to deliver her that day.

Something Wrong

I arrived at the hospital about 1:00 in the afternoon. Robin was in the shower, which was not a good sign. Hot showers were the only thing she had found that helped relieve the pain, other than narcotics. She would take four or five hot showers a day whenever she was sick. Robin came out of the shower and she said, "Mom, there's something wrong. I hurt everywhere. My feet hurt. My hands hurt. Everything hurts. And it started when they hung that bag of stuff there." She pointed to a bag hanging on the IV pole. The only way I can describe it is to say that it looked like a melted chocolate milkshake, sort of like a protein drink. I looked at it and on every corner it said, "Not for IV Use"—and it was hooked to her PICC line, which of course is an IV. And I did not think to question it. I didn't ask anything about it.

Robin called the nurse and asked, "Can you tell my mom what the plan is?" And the nurse said, "Well, we have started her TPN and we are going to keep her in the hospital until she's 37 weeks and wean her off the narcotics because we think that's what is wrong with her. She is getting too many narcotics."

I was a little dubious but I said, "Okay, if that's what we need to do, that's what we'll do." But Robin was so uncomfortable. She asked the nurse why she was in so much pain and the nurse said, "Well, it's because we are not giving you as much pain medicine. You're just anxious and you need to relax." She got her some Vistaril for anxiety. Again, I didn't question it. I went along with them.

Robin tried to rest. She just hurt so much, but they wouldn't give her any more pain medicine. She had been hooked up to a fetal monitor earlier that morning and the strip was still on the monitor. I looked at it, and from the tracing it looked like the baby was asleep. It wasn't very reactive, but because Robin was on narcotics that wasn't surprising. This was another reason the nurse had said that they wanted to keep Robin in the hospital, because the baby's fetal monitor strip wasn't reactive, even though it obviously wasn't going to be if Robin was on narcotics. But again, I didn't question it.

"You've Got to Fix Me"

I had dropped Jerick off at daycare before coming to the hospital, but I had to pick him up at 5:00 p.m. I told Robin, "I've got to go pick up Jerick, but I'll be back when Jeremy gets home from work." I got Jerick and went to their house. I was waiting for Jeremy to get home, when Robin called. She said, "Mom, I need you to come back. They've done something wrong."

I called Jeremy and said, "You need to come home now. They've done something at the hospital and we need to go back there." I got to the hospital about 6:00 p.m. When I walked in the room Robin was on a heart monitor and she had on a facemask with oxygen. She looked at me, and tears just rolled down her cheeks. She said, "Mom, I'm so scared."

I said, "It'll be okay. They're going to take good care of you. We just need to take care of you." But when I put my hand on her back, you could feel and hear, whenever she breathed, the fluid that was in her lungs.

The nurse came in. I asked her, "Have they checked on the baby?"

She said, "Yes, we ran a fetal monitor strip a while ago. The heart rate was 150." But on the monitor Robin's heart rate was also 150. I'm sure they were picking up Robin's heartbeat rather than the baby's. They should have checked Robin's pulse to make sure. But 150 is a very common baby heart rate, and they just took it at face value.

The OB doctor came in about then. He said, "Robin, I think they gave you too much fluid in the emergency room. We're just going to give you some Lasix and we'll get this taken care of."

And he left. The nurse was still there with me. I said, "Is that all they're going to do? Are they going to do something else? She looks terrible."

I didn't say that loud enough for Robin to hear. But she had a terrible color. Her oxygen saturation was 89. Her heart rate was 150. She was having trouble breathing. I said, "What else are you going to do?"

The nurse said, "We'll get the Lasix. We'll get that started."

About that time Robin's doctor came in, the one who'd been taking care of her and who she worked for. He came over, and he gave her a hug. She said, "Chief, you've got to fix me."

He said, "I will, Robin. I'll take care of you." He asked the nurse, "How much of that stuff did she get?"

I hadn't even noticed it when I walked in at 6:00 p.m., but the brown-looking bag was not hanging on the pole any more. She just had a transparent saline solution hanging. The nurse showed the doctor on the computer how much of the brown-looking solution she had been given. He said, "Okay." He ordered Robin more Lasix, and he wanted her to have BiPAP (bilevel positive airway pressure) to help improve her breathing. So the respiratory technician came down and hooked up the BiPAP. She started feeling better. Her oxygen saturation came up to around 93% and she felt more comfortable.

The OB doctor came back in. He said, "Let's check on the baby." He listened for a while and he didn't hear anything. He said, "Let's get the ultrasound." He looked with the ultrasound for a while and he didn't say anything. I looked at it and I didn't see the baby's heartbeat. I could see the baby, because I have looked at a lot of ultrasounds, but I didn't see a heartbeat.

He said, "We need to get the big ultrasound machine down here, to really take a look." And he left.

I walked outside the room. The nurse came out. I asked her, "Did you see a heartbeat?"

The nurse said, "Well, you know, it's not a very good ultrasound machine. It just basically tells us the position of the baby. We're going to get the big machine down here to look again." I said, "Okay."

So they got the big ultrasound machine, and the OB doctor sat at the foot of her bed and he looked for a while. Robin watched the monitor and then she looked at me and she said, "Mom, is she dead?" I said, "Yes, Robin, I believe she is."

And I said, "But we can deal with that, Robin. We just need to take care of you right now." The OB doctor said, "That's right, Robin. You just need to listen to your mom." And he left. He never said anything about the baby or the lack of heartbeat.

A Higher Level

A short time later Robin's doctor came back in. He checked on Robin and then he said to me, "I want to talk to you out in the hall."

I went out into the hall with him. The OB doctor was there. Robin's doctor said, "I think we need to get her to a higher level of care. We have called LifeFlight and we're going to transfer her. But I think it's probably better for us to intubate her here than for them to have to do it in the helicopter."

In my mind, I was thinking, "Okay, we lost the baby. We'll deal with that. Robin is just going to be in another hospital for a few extra days." It never entered my mind that she wouldn't be okay. It just never occurred to me.

We went back in and he told Robin what they wanted to do. And she agreed that we needed to do something different. They called anesthesia to come intubate her.

About that time, her husband Jeremy arrived. Both the doctors were busy and I said, "You guys work on Robin and make sure she's okay. I'll go talk to Jeremy."

I went out and I told him. I said, "Jeremy, the baby's dead, and Robin is so sick that they're going to transfer her. LifeFlight is on its way and they're going to send her out."

I stayed with him a little bit, and then headed back to Robin's room. They stopped me outside the door and said, "You can't go in there."

I said, "That's my daughter in there! I can go wherever I want. I'm going back in there."

They said, "No, you can't go back in there."

I could hear through the door that they were talking about bicarb and epinephrine, and I knew they were coding her. The head nurse came out; I think she was coming out to get something. I stopped her and said, "You guys need to come out here and tell me what is going on. Somebody needs to come out and tell me now."

They took us down to a little room down the hall. They said, "Somebody will come in and talk to you."

Robin's doctor came in. He said, "Well, we've called a cardiologist to come in, but he's not in house. He's on his way in."

They had put in a pacemaker. Without the pacemaker, her heart rate was a slow 30. Even with the pacemaker, they weren't getting any peripheral pulses, so her heart was not pumping enough blood to her brain.

I told him, "Okay, stop. Stop right now. You cannot be talking about one of my girls that way. You need to get back in there and you need to fix her, because this cannot be happening."

He left. He was gone for a few minutes. He came back in and he opened the door. I looked at him and I just turned my back on him.

I said, "Can you keep her alive until her sisters get here to say good-bye?"

He said, "No, I don't think I can."

I said, "I want to see her." They pronounced her dead at 8:36 p.m., 3 days after Jerick's third birthday.

A Tubing Misconnection

The nurse had erroneously given Robin an enteral feed, a thick mixture like a nutritional shake, in her intravenous PICC line. Enteral solution is suitable only for feeding via the gastrointestinal tract, usually through a feeding tube. This error ultimately caused the death of Robin and the baby.

The origin of the error was a little mysterious. A bag of enteral feed with Robin's name on it had been delivered to the unit. The delivery came from the dietary department, because enteral feed was considered a food at that hospital and was dispensed through the dietary department. The total parenteral solution (TPN) that Robin was supposed to have received was considered an IV medication and would have come from the hospital pharmacy. To complicate matters, the hospital had just introduced a new computer system, and they still were hand-writing orders for the secretary to put into the computer. The order for the enteral feeding bag was time-stamped and name-stamped by the unit secretary, but the secretary said she had not put the order in. There were no written physician orders for either the enteral solution or the TPN.

The hospital policy was that two nurses check the label and the ingredients against the order before it was given to the patient. But in this case there was no order, and the nurse did not have a second nurse check it with her and did not scan the bar code on the medication. The nurse knew that the plan was for Robin to get TPN, so that's what she assumed the bag was, even though it looked nothing like TPN.

Typically, a bag of enteral solution comes from the manufacturer attached to a tube that will only fit a feeding tube, not an IV. But not all manufacturers make it that way. In Robin's case, the bag came without tubing. So the nurse got some IV tubing off the shelf, spiked the bag with the tubing, and put the tubing on an IV infusion pump. The enteral solution was too thick to run on its own, so the nurse set the infusion pump to 200 mL an hour and connected it to Robin's PICC line. A PICC line sits right at the arch of the aorta, so the feeding was dumping right into her heart, and it had such a high fat content that everything was clogging up. That's why her feet hurt so much, because all the little vessels in her feet—everything—were just clogging up with fat.

The policy at the hospital was that the nutritionist would see every patient before the patients were started on TPN. The nutritionist was going through the charts and the nurse said, "We've got the

TPN started." This in itself was a policy violation. The nutritionist said, "No, she's not on TPN; there's no order for it." It was then that they noticed the mistake. The enteral feeds were started at 11:00 a.m. and they were stopped around 5:00 p.m. The nurse never realized there was anything wrong until that moment.

Conclusion

The nurse lost her job at the hospital and surrendered her license under a plea agreement that allowed her license to be reinstated after 8 months. When she got her license back, she went to work for the OB doctor involved in Robin's case.

The hospital administration started using the closed tubing system so nurses did not have to attach the tubing, and they made enteral feedings the responsibility of the pharmacy rather than the dietary department, so that a licensed healthcare professional would be checking the orders. They also did a lot of education to try to make their nurses aware of tubing misconnections.

I started talking about tubing misconnections to everyone I could get to listen. I have been part of an international group working on new standards, but change is coming much more slowly than I would like. As a nurse, I have changed my practice about patients and families asking questions. I know that sometimes it can feel as though families are questioning your ability and authority. But if there is something that doesn't look right, families should ask the question. If the nurse sees something that doesn't look right, the nurse should question it. If you don't get a good answer, question it again. Keep questioning until you get a resolution. I will go to my grave wishing that I had done that for Robin and Addison.

Case Discussion

Delivering modern healthcare requires many tubing connections that can lead to errors with medical tubing or catheters. This problem has been recognized since the 1970s. The interchangeable Luer lock used in the connection of medical components and accessories has allowed for many misconnections every year, not just of IVs, but also other devices, including blood pressure cuffs and endotracheal tubes (Guenter et al., 2008; U.S. Food and Drug Administration, 2012). Experts believe the only real solution is the redesign of tubing connections to eliminate the possibility of connections between incompatible systems (Vockley, 2011).

Of the many connection errors that occur, the misconnection of an enteral feeding system with an IV tube is especially feared because the resulting introduction of high-fat solution into the bloodstream is not reversible and the outcome for the patient is likely to be death. Like other tubing misconnections, enteral misconnections are usually the result of nursing error, and the legal and professional consequences for nurses can be severe, as they were for Robin's nurse. Researchers who study tubing misconnections, however, view them as primarily a human factors problem, an unconscious slip that occurs as the practitioner automatically performs a routine task (Simmons & Graves, 2008). Human factors, or human factors engineering, is "the discipline that attempts to identify and address safety problems that arise due to the interaction between people, technology, and work environments" (Agency for Healthcare Research and Quality, 2012).

The actual historical frequency of enteral tubing misconnections is not known, but a 2011 review of the literature showed more than 116 cases of enteral misconnection documented in medical journals (Simmons, Symes, Guenter, & Graves, 2011). An international collaboration, in which Robin Lowe's mother Glenda is included, has been underway for many years to develop International Standard Organization (ISO) standards for manufacturers of tubing connectors. Partly in recognition of the seriousness of the problem, the first connectors to be produced under the revised standards are part of a new enteral feeding system that cannot be connected to incompatible delivery systems like intravenous tubing. The change to the new standards is taking place in phases, with transitional connectors available so that facilities can continue to use existing stocks of tubing. Use of the new connectors will not be mandatory in any American state except California, although interchangeable connectors will gradually cease to be available as manufacturers adopt the revised ISO standards (Global Enteral Device Supplier Association, 2014; The Joint Commission, 2014).

Questions

1. Discuss the chain of events and mistakes that led to the death of Robin and her baby. At what point could the pending disaster have been stopped? What processes could be put in place to prevent such an event from occurring?

2. The most significant change that the hospital made was to stop buying enteral feeding solution that came without the tubing attached. Research human factors theory and discuss the human factors issues that arise with tubing misconnections. How can forcing functions like the anticipated move to specialized connectors improve the situation?

3. Glenda Rodgers blames herself for not asking more questions when her daughter was in the hospital. She feels that, as an experienced obstetrical nurse, she should have caught what was going on and been able to put a stop to it. Yet stories of healthcare professionals being unable to stop adverse events from happening to their own family members are common. Why do you think that healthcare professionals may feel helpless to prevent errors when they become a patient or have a family member who is a patient?

4. Research the concept of *just culture*, and discuss how you think it applies in this case. What should the consequences have been for the nurse who caused the tubing misconnection?

5. As the rollout of new tubing connector standards began, the American accrediting agency The Joint Commission issued Sentinel Event Alert No. 53 to help healthcare facilities deal with the transition. Why do you think The Joint Commission considered this to be necessary? What unintended consequences should healthcare professionals be vigilant for when changes take place in practice and technology?

6. Which of the core competencies for health professions are most relevant for this case? Why?

References

Agency for Healthcare Research and Quality. (2012). Human factors engineering. AHRQ PSNet. Available at: http://www.psnet.ahrq.gov /primer.aspx?primerID=20.

Guenter, P., Hicks, R., Simmons, D., Crowley, J., Croteau, R., Gosnell, C., Pratt, N. G., & Vanderveen, T. W. (2008). Enteral feeding misconnections: A consortium position statement. *Joint Commission Journal on Quality and Patient Safety*, *34*(5), 285–292.

Global Enteral Device Supplier Association. (2014). New ENFit Connectors Due in US, Canada, Puerto Rico in 2014; Europe and other markets anticipate to begin transition in 2015. Stay Connected 2014. Available at: http://www.stayconnected2014.org/get-ready.html

Simmons, D., & Graves, K. (2008). Tubing misconnections—a systems failure with human factors: Lessons for nursing practice. *Urologic Nursing*, *28*(6), 460–464.

Simmons, D., Symes, L., Guenter, P., & Graves, K. (2011). Tubing misconnections: Normalization of deviance. *Nutrition in Clinical Practice*, *26*(3), 286–293.

The Joint Commission. (2014, August 20). Managing risk during transiton to new ISO tubing connector standards. Sentinel Event Alert 53. Available at: http://www.jointcommission.org/sea_issue_53/

U.S. Food and Drug Administration. (2012). Tubing and Luer misconnections: Preventing dangerous medical errors. Available at: http:// www.fda.gov/MedicalDevices/Safety/AlertsandNotices/Tubingand-LuerMisconnections/default.htm.

Vockley, M. (2011). Dangerous connections: Healthcare community tackles tubing risks. *Biomedical Instrumentation & Technology*, *45*(6), 426–428, 430–422, 434.

Death Despite Known Drug Allergy

The Story of Zoya (Australia)

Farah Magrabi, Dale Ford, Diana Arachi,
and Helena Williams

Editors' Note

Zoya,[1] a 36-year-old factory worker, lived in a suburb 25 km southwest of Sydney, Australia. She had a history of allergic reactions resulting in previous admissions to local hospitals. In July 1998, she was treated for an allergic reaction to Septrin, a sulfonamide antibiotic containing sulfamethoxazole and trimethoprim; later, in September 2004, she presented with a widespread itchy rash resulting from an allergic reaction to cephalexin, a cephalosporin antibiotic.

Hospital records indicated that she had an allergy to penicillin. Her primary care records noted that she was allergic to Ibilex, (brand name for cephalexin); Ilosone (a brand name for erythromycin), another antibiotic; and sulfur-based antibiotics. In other words, Zoya suffered from pan-allergies to multiple antibiotics. Her family was well aware of her allergies, especially to sulfa-containing medications.

LEARNING OBJECTIVES

After completing this case study, you will be able to:

1. Discuss how clinical decision support tools within electronic prescribing software has the potential to prevent medication errors and adverse drug events.

[1] Names have been changed to protect the privacy of those involved in this case.

2. Create a strategy for ensuring the role of patients and consumers as participants in the care process and in safeguarding against medical error.

3. Identify the potential risks of hybrid paper and electronic medical records.

A Visit to Her Regular Primary Care Clinic

Zoya worked at the same factory for 5 years. On a Monday morning in the middle of a cold winter she returned home after a night shift by 8 a.m., feeling ill. When asked by John, her partner, what was wrong, she explained that she had a sore ear and would be making an appointment with the doctor. John had been in a relationship with Zoya for many years. Zoya's right ear had been bothering her for about 3 days. As she seemed fine and was not in any great pain, John went to work.

Zoya booked an appointment with a local primary care clinic, the Get Well Clinic. This clinic was not her first choice. Her preferred family general practitioner (GP) worked at another clinic 2 km away. She had rung them first that morning, but after detailing the nature of her problem she was told that they had no appointments available for the next 3 days.

The Get Well Clinic was a very busy, fully accredited clinic with many doctors. Zoya had frequently visited this clinic for the last 10 years, usually when her family GP had no available appointments. At Get Well it was common for the doctors to see certain patients regularly as well as patients who might attend the clinic to see any doctor available on the day.

On that day Zoya saw Dr. Stanley, a very experienced 70-year-old physician. He was a registered GP who had worked in the medical profession for almost 50 years and had practiced as an associate at Get Well for the last few years. He usually worked around 20 hours per week, mostly on weekdays, but also sometimes assisted the clinic on weekends. He was highly esteemed by his patients and colleagues.

The Consultation

Dr. Stanley saw Zoya shortly after 11:00 a.m. During the consultation Zoya complained of a severe earache that was affecting the entire right side of her face.[2] She said that the pain had been bothering her for 3 days. Ear pain is a common reason for primary care consultations and is the 20th most frequent complaint cited by patients. GPs typically see 14 patients with ear pain in every 1000 consultations (Britt et al., 2010). Zoya also told Dr. Stanley that she was a smoker.

Dr. Stanley took her history and examined both of Zoya's ears with an otoscope.[3] He noticed that the outer ear canal was very inflamed on the right side. The middle ear appeared normal, and he made the diagnosis of otitis externa, an inflammation of the outer ear and ear canal. He did not detect any abnormalities when he performed a routine examination of Zoya's abdomen, throat, heart, and lungs with her lying on the examination table. Dr. Stanley's usual practice was to treat otitis externa with topical antibiotic ointments or alternatively with oral medication. Given the severity of Zoya's ear infection, he decided to prescribe the oral antibiotic cefaclor (Ceclor).[4]

Dr. Stanley's usual practice was to check a patient's records for details of any recorded allergies and ask the patient three questions:

1. Are you taking any medications?
2. Are you allergic to anything?
3. And, are you allergic to any medications?

If the patient answered "yes" to any of these questions, he would ask further questions to ascertain what medications the patient was allergic to. Dr. Stanley could not recall more details of his assessment

---

[2] According to MedlinePlus, causes of ear pain include acute ear infection, chronic ear infection, and sinus infection (http://www.nlm.nih.gov/medlineplus/ency/article/003046.htm).

[3] An otoscope is a medical device used to examine the outer ear and middle ear.

[4] Cefaclor is a second-generation cephalosporin antibiotic.

and could not recall his conversation with Zoya in relation to allergies. He later gave evidence that it was not his usual practice to review a patient's previous notes in detail prior to a consultation.

Writing the Prescription

The Get Well Clinic used an electronic system to maintain medical records. The entire medical record was maintained electronically; there were no paper records at this clinic. At the time of Zoya's consultation, the vast majority of GPs (77%) were prescribing electronically, and 54% maintained electronic medical records (i.e., paperless systems offered by commercial clinical software packages that enable practitioners to enter progress notes, write prescriptions, and order laboratory tests, as well as other tasks) (Britt et al., 2010). Most software packages also provide degrees of clinical decision support, such as access to clinical evidence and tools to check for drug allergies as well as drug–drug and drug–disease interactions. The prescriptions were created electronically, and printed copies were given to the patient.

Dr. Stanley was never proficient with the desktop computer in his consultation room. When he started working at the clinic he was given some basic training on the use of electronic medical records. He was aware about the procedure for entering the details of a consultation (clinical progress notes). He knew that the electronic medical record allowed him to go back and review the details of previous consultations and that it contained details of medications prescribed to the patient and any allergies that had been reported. His usual practice when seeing a patient was to first obtain a history from the patient as to the presenting complaint, conduct an examination, and then provide or recommend necessary treatment. When the patient left the room, he would make a note of the consultation before the next patient came in. It was not his practice to enter notes on the computer while the patient was in the room.

He gave Zoya a handwritten prescription for Ceclor, (a brand name for cefaclor), at a dose of 375 mg to be taken twice per day for 5 days. He also provided her with a medical work certificate for 1 day off work. The consultation lasted about 10 minutes. After Zoya left the room, he immediately made his consultation note on the computer at 11:17 a.m. He failed to notice the allergy information on the screen when entering his clinical progress notes into the electronic record. Contrary to his normal practice, he did not review his notes to look for a reference to drug allergies.

The Fatal Dose

Zoya took the prescription to a local pharmacist to have the medication dispensed. It appears that the medication was dispensed without question. She then returned home and took the first prescribed dose. Shortly after midday John returned home to find Zoya unconscious, lying sideways across the bottom of the bed on her side, with her legs over the edge of the bed, and looking red with a number of welts on her body. Her face was swollen and she was not breathing. He shouted her name, but she did not respond and her lips were blue. When he could not rouse her, he called the emergency services at 12:18 p.m. His call was dispatched to the ambulance service, and they talked him through the process of resuscitation (CPR). He had no formal training in CPR.

An ambulance arrived at 12:26 p.m., and the paramedics noted that Zoya was in full cardiac arrest. She had no pulse and was not breathing. The paramedics commenced CPR and continued to work at the scene for almost an hour. Adrenaline and atropine were administered, and she was intubated and transferred to a hospital. A box of medication labeled cefaclor was found by the paramedics on the lounge room table with one tablet missing from the blister pack.

Zoya arrived at the local hospital at 1:29 p.m. and was admitted to the intensive care unit (ICU) in critical condition and requiring ongoing life support. Over the next 2 days her condition deteriorated, with a loss of spontaneous respiration and the onset of hypotension and hypothermia. On Wednesday at 9:59 a.m. a perfusion scan was conducted that showed Zoya's cerebral perfusion was absent, which indicated that she had no blood perfusing her brain.

Events beginning on a Monday

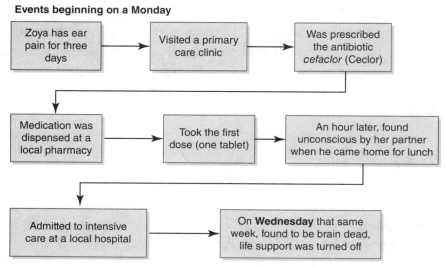

Figure 19-1. Zoya's Story

At 10:58 a.m. the doctors stated that she satisfied the criteria for brain death. She was extubated, all medications were stopped, and she was pronounced dead at 1:07 p.m.

Figure 19-1 summarizes the events that occurred.

The Aftermath

Zoya had suffered an immediate anaphylactic[5] reaction most likely mediated by IgE[6]. Allergic reactions are characterized by the development of systemic hemodynamic collapse within 1–2 hours of medication administration (Antibiotic Expert Group, 2010). Anaphylaxis to cephalosporin antibiotics is rare (estimated at 0.0001–0.1%), but it can be fatal (Kelkar & Li, 2001). In Australia, there are approximately 15 anaphylaxis-related deaths each year (6.4 deaths per 10 million population) (Liew et al., 2009). Of the 112 anaphylaxis-related deaths

[5] Anaphylaxis is a rapidly developing serious allergic reaction that may cause death. It is commonly caused by insect stings, food, and medication, and results in an itchy rash, throat swelling, and low blood pressure.

[6] An IgE-mediated reaction is an abnormal response of the immune system to a medication.

between 1997 and 2005, 57% were linked to medications. Most deaths have occurred in adults older than 55 years of age. Cefaclor is a moderate-spectrum cephalosporin antibiotic and is generally not recommended for the treatment of otitis externa by the Australian guidelines for general practice (Antibiotic Expert Group, 2010). Moreover, cefaclor is contraindicated in patients with a prior allergic reaction to a cephalosporin or a history of severe or immediate (IgE-mediated) allergic reaction to penicillins or carbapenems (including urticaria, anaphylaxis, or interstitial nephritis, DRESS syndrome, or Stevens-Johnson syndrome) (Rossi, 2011). The Australian guidelines state that a cephalosporin, a carbapenem, or penicillin should not be given if there is a clear or vague history of an immediate (IgE-mediated) reaction to penicillin (Antibiotic Expert Group, 2010; Rossi, 2011). It is not known if Dr. Stanley had access to or considered any clinical guidelines during the time he examined the patient.

Dr. Stanley *later* became aware that Zoya had allergies to Ibilex (cephalexin), Ilosone (erythromycin), and sulfa-based drugs, and this sensitivity was noted in Zoya's medical record. He had failed to observe the entry in her electronic record that indicated her allergies. He could not recall an alert on the screen in relation to patient allergies. Rather, he recalled that it was necessary to scroll back to the top of the record to check for this information. He was later advised that information relating to allergies appears on the screen at the top of every patient record. He knew that cefaclor was similar to cephalexin in that it belonged to the same group of antibiotics called cephalosporins and that patients who were allergic to cephalosporins can suffer a variety of reactions. He said later that had he known that Zoya had an allergy to cephalexin he would not have prescribed cefaclor.

Dr. Stanley had no previous performance issues with his practice. Six days after Zoya's death he resigned from the Get Well Clinic, never resumed medical practice, and let his medical registration lapse. He accepted that the information about allergies would likely have been on the screen at the time he typed the note of his consultation with Zoya. As a consequence of Zoya's death he became depressed and suffered considerably. He demonstrated considerable guilt, shame, and self-reproach about the effect and outcomes of his treatment of Zoya.

Conclusion

The tragic outcome was over in 2 days. A simple antibiotic allergy was not identified during a routine consultation for a commonly treated condition. A prescribing error occurred and propagated through the system. It was not detected when writing the prescription due to the use of a hybrid medical record system whereby the prescription was written on paper and the progress notes were entered electronically after the patient had left the room. The error was also not detected when the medication was dispensed by the pharmacy, and the patient died from anaphylaxis after taking one tablet.

Case Discussion

Treatment of Otitis Externa with an Oral Antibiotic

Dr. Stanley's decision to prescribe an antibiotic may not have been appropriate. Oral antibiotics are not generally recommended for otitis externa (Antibiotic Expert Group, 2010). The main issue surrounding the management of this condition is the choice between topical and systemic treatment and indications for antibiotic drops. A trial of common treatments for acute otitis externa in primary care demonstrated that applying steroid drops in combination with acetic acid or antibiotics improves outcomes with a reduction in duration of symptoms when compared to acetic acid drops alone (Van Balen, Smit, Zuithoff, & Verheij, 2003). Another study showed a lower rate of persistent infection and subsequent consultation after treatment with topical steroids with or without antibiotics over oral therapy (Rowlands et al., 2001).

Even if treatment with an oral antibiotic was justified, cefaclor was not an appropriate choice for Zoya given her allergies and history of allergic reactions. This medication is contraindicated in patients with a known allergy to the cephalosporin group of antibiotics or who have previously experienced a major allergy to penicillin (GP2U Telehealth Pty. Ltd., 2012). The product information for cefaclor (GP2U Telehealth Pty. Ltd., 2012) states that anaphylaxis to oral penicillin or cephalosporins is "more likely to occur in individuals with a history of penicillin hypersensitivity and/or a history of sensitivity to multiple allergens." Moreover, there are reports of "individuals with a history of penicillin/cephalosporin hypersensitivity who have experienced severe reactions when treated with a penicillin/cephalosporin." It is not clear if Dr. Stanley checked Zoya's current medications and known allergies and adverse drug reactions, as recommended by the Australian standards for general practice (Royal Australian College of General Practitioners, 2010).

Data Quality

A number of problems were apparent with the allergy information in Zoya's hospital and clinic medical records:

- Allergy information maintained by both the hospital and clinic was incomplete. The hospital had no record of the erythromycin allergy, and the penicillin allergy was not recorded in the clinic records.
- In both medical records, allergies were specified by brand names (e.g., Ibilex, Ilosone, Septrin), rather than their generic names (i.e., cephalexin, erythromycin, sulfamethoxazole and trimethoprim, respectively).
- The hospital discharge records from Zoya's previous adverse drug reactions were not available at either of the primary care clinics she visited (i.e., the Get Well Clinic or her family GP).

Procedures for Use of Hybrid and Paper Medical Records

Medical records can be maintained in paper form, electronically, or in a hybrid medical record system. A hybrid medical record system, the most common type in healthcare systems today, is where a mix of paper and electronic media are used to maintain the medical records for a single patient. For example, a GP might prescribe electronically and use a paper record to maintain the progress notes. At the time of this event, 29% of Australian GPs used a hybrid medical record system and 65% maintained medical records electronically (Britt et al., 2010). In many paperless practices, test results (e.g., pathology, imaging) and consultation letters are received on paper and need to be scanned into the electronic records system, often by administrative staff. Although letters and results are usually read and acknowledged by clinical staff (e.g., GPs) before being uploaded into a patient's medical record, changes to the patient's past medical histories, known clinical conditions, and/or allergies are not necessarily always updated systematically as new letters are noted.

The workflow adopted by Dr. Stanley transformed the paperless system at Get Well into a hybrid record system whereby he used the electronic system to record progress notes and wrote prescriptions on paper. The Australian standards for general practice, recognizing the risks of hybrid and paper records, recommend a "note in each system to improve the continuity of hybrid systems" and suggest that practices with hybrid patient health record systems "work toward the electronic recording of at least allergies and medications" (Royal Australian College of General Practitioners, 2010). The specific risks of this scenario where progress notes are maintained electronically and prescriptions are generated on paper is not highlighted. However, it is clearly stated that "where a practice uses a hybrid health record system, it is particularly important that the allergy status of the patient is recorded in the same system that is used for prescription writing."

Problems with Decision Support in the Clinical Software Package

The use of a clinical decision support system within electronic prescribing software has the potential to prevent medication errors and adverse drug events. However, Dr. Stanley's clinical oversight could not be detected by the drug–allergy software utility within the clinical software package for two reasons:

1. *Lack of a hard stop.* The clinical decision support system did not have a "hard stop" feature. Prescriptions could be created without recording any information about the patient's allergies in the medical record. A safe forcing function design would require the doctor to record known allergies or confirm no known allergies. That is, it would have a hard stop—it would not allow the doctor to continue his workflow by creating a prescription without recording allergy information.

2. *Configuration of decision support rules for generating prescribing alerts.* In general, an allergy can be specified by the generic name of a medication, its brand name, or by the medication class. In Zoya's case, an allergy to the brand Ibilex was noted in her medical record and visible on the screen when her file was opened up. Had Dr. Stanley used a computer to generate the prescription for cefaclor during the consultation the allergy to Ibilex would have been displayed on the screen. But, contrary to expectations, a pop-up alert warning him about Zoya's allergy was not displayed by the software package. The rules of the decision support system in this particular instance were configured to go off only for the medication specified in the allergy entry (i.e., for the medication Ibilex, a specific brand of cephalexin, and not for all cephalosporin antibiotics). Nor would the alert be activated if Keflex, another brand for cephalexin, was prescribed. To detect Dr. Stanley's prescribing error the decision support system in this particular software required an allergy to be specifically entered by *class* for all cephalosporin antibiotics.

At the Pharmacy: A Missed Opportunity to Detect a Prescribing Error

Community pharmacies could play an important role in detecting potential adverse events associated with medications. There was no information about what transpired at the pharmacy and the process in which the antibiotics for Zoya were dispensed. It was not clear if a pharmacist or an assistant dispensed the medication, and many questions remain unresolved:

- What happened at the pharmacy?
- Who dispensed the antibiotic? A pharmacist or a pharmacy assistant?
- In line with Australian standards for pharmacy dispensing, did the person dispensing the antibiotic ask Zoya about any suspected and known adverse drug reactions, precautions, and contraindications when dispensing the medication (Pharmaceutical Society of Australia, 2010)?
- Did the pharmacy software package used for dispensing Zoya's medications have a feature to record and alert the pharmacist about Zoya's potential allergic reactions?

Questions

1. Human factors research has taught about the need for system redundancies. Where was the redundancy in the system? Identify redundant processes or components in the system that can detect and mitigate the effects of prescribing errors.

2. Evaluate the effectiveness of the clinical handover in Zoya's care between the multiple GPs within the Get Well Clinic, her family GP, and the local hospital.

3. Compare and contrast the advantages and disadvantages of health systems with high levels of continuity of care. Using this lens, what part do you think continuity of care played in this case?

4. What actions can be taken by the organizations, professional bodies, and individuals to prevent such incidents in future? Discuss specifically actions that could have been taken by one or more of the following:

   a. Zoya

   b. Zoya's family

   c. The Get Well Clinic

   d. The family GP

   e. The pharmacy

    f. The local hospital

    g. National health, patient safety, and general practice training and representative organizations

5. Discuss the risks of a hybrid medical records system. How would you ensure safety of the work practice adopted by Dr. Stanley whereby he accessed and updated the computer record only after the patient had left the room, particularly with regard to the following?

    a. Review of patient records before and during the consultation.

    b. Recording of prescriptions and medical certificates that were generated on paper.

6. What are the implications of this case for training? Discuss requirements for training in the safe use of clinical software.

7. Examine how allergies are recorded and evaluate the display of allergy information in prescribing and dispensing software. Discuss the role of software standards.

8. How might you design a pharmacy software system to minimize the risk of medication errors? How might the following special populations affect the use and design of pharmacy software systems?

    a. Residents in an aged care facility

    b. A community with a language other than English

    c. Populations with poor health literacy

9. What role did health literacy limitations potentially play in this case?

10. What is the role of patients or consumers and their caregivers in health care? Will they be expected to play a different role and take more responsibility for their health care, especially with the advent of personal health records that all citizens can access and maintain electronically?

11. How might personal or shared electronic health records help in preventing adverse events?

12. Which of the core competencies for health professions are most relevant for this case? Why?

Acknowledgments

We wish to thank Professor Enrico Coiera for his constructive feedback.

References

Antibiotic Expert Group. (2010). *Therapeutic guidelines: Antibiotic. Version 14*. Melbourne: Therapeutic Guidelines Ltd.

Britt, H., Miller, G. C., Charles, J., Henderson, J., Bayram, C., Pan, Y., . . . Fahridin, S. (2010). General practice activity in Australia 2009–10. Cat. no. GEP 27. Canberra: Australian Institute of Health and Welfare.

GP2U Telehealth Pty. Ltd. (2012). Ceclor (cefaclor) marketed product information. Available at: http://www.pbs.gov.au/meds%2Fpi%2Faspceclo11109.pdf.

Kelkar, P. S., & Li, J. T. (2001). Cephalosporin allergy. *New England Journal of Medicine, 345*, 804–809.

Liew, W. K., Williamson, E., & Tang, M. L. (2009). Anaphylaxis fatalities and admissions in Australia. *Jounral of Allergy and Clinical Immunolology, 123*(2), 434–442.

Pharmaceutical Society of Australia. (2010). Professional practice standards (version 4). Available at: http://www.psa.org.au/supporting-practice/professional-practice-standards/version-4.

Rossi, S. (Ed.). (2011). *Australian medicines handbook* (11th ed.). Adelaide: AMH Pty Ltd.

Rowlands, S., Devalia, H., Smith, C., Hubbard, R., & Dean, A. (2001). Otitis externa in UK general practice: A survey using the UK General Practice Research Database. *British Journal of General Practice, 51*(468), 533–538.

Royal Australian College of General Practitioners. (2010). Standards for general practices (4th ed.). Available at: http://www.psa.org.au/download/standards/professional-practice-standards-v4.pdf.

Van Balen, F. A., Smit, W. M., Zuithoff, N. P., & Verheij, T. J. (2003). Clinical efficacy of three common treatments in acute otitis externa in primary care: Randomised controlled trial. *BMJ, 327*(7425), 1201–1205.

The Trial Meant for You: The Lifelong Medical Journey of a Child with a Complex Congenital Condition

The Story of Kirsten Morrise (United States)

Lisa Morrise and Kirsten Morrise

Editors' Note

Lisa Morrise defines herself as an accidental advocate. Originally trained in broadcasting, she was a National Association of Broadcasters Student of the Year when studying journalism at the University of Kansas. But after her marriage, the birth of three children with differing special needs led her down a different path.

By far the most medically complex of Lisa's children was her daughter Kirsten, who was born with a genetic condition called Pierre Robin sequence. The term sequence *denotes a series of anomalies stemming from a single malformation. In Pierre Robin sequence, the initial defect is a jaw that fails to develop normally before birth. This leads to a severely recessed chin, a cleft palate, and a tongue that falls back into the throat. The result is usually a compromised airway and problems in sucking and swallowing (Breugem & Mink Van Der Molen, 2009). In some cases, the child's jaw catches up in growth after birth if the child is supported with a feeding tube and careful positioning (always face down) to avoid obstructing the airway. Children like Kirsten, with a more severe defect, can require repeated surgical and medical intervention to restore normal facial structure and a functioning airway (Shinghal & Tewfik, 2008).*

Kirsten, now a young adult, has undergone dozens of surgeries and procedures. Her mother Lisa left broadcasting years ago to devote herself to her daughter's care. As part of her involvement with Kirsten's health care, Lisa joined her hospital's patient advisory council and embarked on a second career as a healthcare consultant. Lisa and Kirsten recount the experiences and lessons of a lifetime of medical intervention, beginning with the events surrounding Kirsten's birth and ending with Lisa's role as a patient leader.

LEARNING OBJECTIVES

After completing this case study, you will be able to:

1. Discuss the potential cognitive biases that can arise in providing care for complex conditions and strategies to overcome these biases.

2. Evaluate the implications of routine training for special circumstances in neonatal resuscitation.

3. List the most important criteria to be considered in forming a patient/family advisory council.

Kirsten's Birth

In contrast to my first two pregnancies, in which I did not have enough amniotic fluid, during Kirsten's pregnancy I had way too much. At 16 weeks into the pregnancy I was put onto bed rest due to high blood pressure. My obstetrician wanted to deliver Kirsten early, but amniocentesis at both 35 and 37 weeks showed no surfactant in the amniotic fluid. Because surfactant is necessary for infant survival and proper pulmonary functioning, this was interpreted to mean that the baby's lungs were not developed. In retrospect they should have known she had challenges, even in utero.

Finally, at 38 weeks my labor was induced with Pitocin. The induction really did not go very well. The anesthesia resident tried and failed three times to place an epidural block; although it was not my intent, this was to be a "natural" birth. As I labored, the nurses kept turning up the Pitocin, because the contractions were not showing up on the monitor. Even as I writhed in pain, they refused to believe me when I told them I was experiencing effective contractions. As a consequence, they increased the Pitocin up to twice as high as it had been in my previous induced delivery. When they finally broke my water and inserted an internal monitor, the contractions registered higher than the machine could measure, and Kirsten's heart was slowing with each contraction. The nurses hurried to turn off the Pitocin. Kirsten was delivered almost immediately and whisked to the other side of the room for resuscitation. They really had to work on her. I had no idea what was going on.

They took Kirsten out of the room and put her in the newborn nursery (not in the NICU). Two hours later, at about 8:00 at night, still woozy from the ordeal, I was wheeled to the nursery to meet my baby. A resident physician was cradling her head in one hand while attempting to feed her with a special bottle with the other. Kirsten was on her back. She was blue, her sides were retracting, and she had no monitors attached. The resident casually turned his head to address me, saying, "So, do clefts run in your family?"

No one had told me up to that point that there was anything wrong with my daughter. I burst into tears. Right then a nurse who had just come on duty said, "She has really never pinked up." She grabbed my baby from the resident and *ran* with her to the newborn intensive care unit. That nurse may well have saved Kirsten's life.

At midnight, 4 hours later, I told them I wanted to hold my baby. A kind nurse took me over to meet my daughter more formally. Kirsten was lying face down on a slanted open crib with monitors and blow-by oxygen. They did not want to tell me what was wrong with her. They just said, "We are not really sure you can hold her; she is having a hard time keeping her oxygen levels up." Eventually I was able to briefly cuddle with Kirsten up on my shoulder. Then the alarms sounded and the nurse put her back in her crib, face down.

The next day I was told that Kirsten had a rare birth defect called Pierre Robin sequence. In a nutshell, Kirsten was born unable to breathe or swallow. She had a recessed lower chin, and her tongue blocked her airway, especially when she was on her back. She also had a complete U-shaped cleft palate—or in other words, no palate at all. This meant that she had extreme difficulties breathing unless she was held face down all the time, even for diaper changes. She was hypoxic the entire first 2 hours of her life, up until that vigilant nurse took her to the intensive care unit. Subsequently, as she has encountered learning disabilities and some cerebral palsy, we suspect that it comes, in part at least, from the 2 hours of oxygen deprivation at the time of her birth.

I was never told that they had made a mistake. I figured it out eventually, but I was never told directly. It took me several years to put all the pieces together and become more aware of what should and should not happen, especially as I had the opportunity to meet other children with a similar birth defect who had also been affected by inappropriate care at birth. Sixteen years later, I went to a dinner for alumni of the newborn intensive care unit. At my table were two nurse educators from the obstetric unit at this hospital. They asked me who my child was and what our experience had been. I told them, thinking of course that no one would remember because it had been 16 years. Instead, they said, "We know who you are." I was shocked. They said, "Ever since your daughter was born, we train every year on Pierre Robin sequence so no one else will experience what you experienced."

Pierre Robin sequence can be detected prenatally, and there are guidelines and processes to follow at birth (American Heart Association in collaboration with the International Liaison Committee on Resuscitation, 2000). Because of my high blood pressure, I was receiving regular ultrasounds and in fact had a biophysical profile done prior to Kirsten's delivery. Even Kirsten's dad and I, both of us nonmedical people, could see on the ultrasound that she had a severely recessed chin. Too much amniotic fluid, no surfactant in the amniotic fluid, and a severely recessed chin—these are all signs of Pierre Robin sequence (Hsieh et al., 1999). Because surfactant was not showing up in my amniocentesis fluid, the doctors focused instead on the concern that Kirsten's lungs were not developed. But surfactant was not showing up because Kirsten could not swallow. The obstruction also meant she could not breathe, so there was no exchange of fluid with her lungs. So when she presented with hypoxia, once they got her oxygen levels up the first time, they relaxed because they figured her lungs were working. They really did not know that this was a baby with a congenital defect.

Kirsten's Surgeries

In the succeeding years, Kirsten has had 41 surgeries. Her first surgery was a lip-tongue adhesion, where the plastic surgeon cut Kirsten's tongue out of her throat and actually grafted it to her lip. A few days after this surgery I read in a cleft palate craniofacial journal what the protocols were for establishing which patients should have lip-tongue adhesion. Kirsten clearly did not qualify. The surgery did not solve her problems with breathing or swallowing. She needed a tracheotomy, which was the alternative treatment. But the plastic surgeon insisted that his surgery had worked, even though clinically it had not. I finally organized a case conference with Kirsten's new ear, nose, and throat surgeon; her pediatrician; and a very outspoken occupational therapist at the table. The other three providers ganged up on the plastic surgeon and said that my child needed a tracheotomy and soon, or she was going to have more problems. When the plastic surgeon was confronted by his colleagues in the room he acquiesced.

Kirsten had the lip-tongue adhesion taken down when she was 6 months old and had a tracheotomy and a gastronomy tube—a G-tube—placed for feeding. She had surgery to repair her cleft palate. She had a surgery to take out the G-tube eventually when she was able to tolerate full feeds. She had surgery to repair the fistulas from the G-tube in her trachea. She had surgeries to build some sinuses because she was born with her sinuses closed off. She continued to have airway problems and was still on continuous breathing support (CPAP) after the tracheotomy was taken down, so she had her adenoids and her tonsils removed. She had bronchoscopies to remove scar tissue where her tracheotomy had been. She had another tracheotomy placed when she was 8 because she was having so much trouble sleeping at night. She needed several liters of oxygen at night, and her airway still would get obstructed. She had nursing care at night from the time she was 2 years old. The nurse would sometimes stagger out in the morning because it had been so difficult to get Kirsten to start breathing again.

At age 12 she had a jaw distraction, which is where they slice open your lower jaw and put screws on either side with a pin between them. A couple of times a day I would turn a screw, just slightly increasing the space. One of the distracters gouged into her ear so we had to stop turning the screw on one side, and Kirsten ended up with a crooked jaw. Then she outgrew her airway and needed to have her upper jaw advanced, for which they did a traditional "break and plate" surgery. When this procedure was performed they fixed her previous jaw distraction surgery and brought everything forward.

The surgeries have not resolved the problem of the compromised airway. Kirsten still struggles to breathe. She has a partially blocked airway in the day due to scar tissue in her trachea, and 100% blockage at night because her tongue still falls back into her airway when she sleeps. She continues to need CPAP when she sleeps. She has just had her third jaw advancement surgery and will need another operation to fix the obstructed trachea. We are hopeful that the third time will be the charm, but we recognize that she may need support for breathing throughout her life. See **Box 20-1** for an interview with Kirsten Morrise on the unique challenges she faces due to her disability.

Conclusion

We have been through a lot over the years, and not all of it was predictable. It is not like there is a knock on your door and the heavenly express drops off the trial that was meant for you. We have

Box 20-1 Unique Challenges: An Interview with Kirsten Morrise

On living with brain injury: I will talk about some of what I deal with related to hypoxic brain injury. For starters I can read. I can read words; my brain just cannot form words into paragraphs. I have a really hard time processing what I read. I have to have most of what I read in audio form so I can comprehend it. I am really good at comprehension; I just cannot pick it up by reading visually. Also, I can write, but it causes my hands a lot of pain. So basically I made it through high school mostly on verbal acuity. I have lower stamina than other kids. When I was little I was the kid who was picked last at kickball. I am also, at times, slower at things. I have a hard time picking up sarcasm. I used to have a lot of trouble picking up on social cues. I had to go to some therapy for that. I have a bad temper sometimes because when you cannot read using the usual cues and you get no sleep because of sleep apnea you are really grumpy. So growing up I was sometimes hard to live with and that required behavioral intervention as well.

On the effects of actions on others: I would not take any of this back because I have had so many great experiences and I have done things that everyone had thought were impossible for me. That does not mean that this had to happen. It did not have to happen, and it is very challenging to deal with. If people had just taken the steps necessary to make sure that my coming into this world was assured to be at the best quality possible then my life maybe could have been more "normal." Take the nurse who left me unattended for 2 hours without oxygen. He made one mistake. In his mind maybe it was not so big, but it affected my life. I would tell nurses and healthcare staff, "Be more cautious when you do things; be more careful and pay attention. Don't be afraid to act in a patient's interest even if in the short haul you get scrutinized for it."

On adversity: If bad things did not happen we would not be able to appreciate the good things. We need to have trials in order to appreciate blessings.

On courage: Being courageous is not about what you go through; it is about how you choose to respond to it. I had to write an essay on courage for my church and I looked up the definition. It said, "Courage is the attitude you display while enduring a trial. It is about the choices that you make that reflect your attitude." If someone goes through a trial, but they do not want to get up and do something about it, they just want to use it as an excuse to lie on the couch—that is not courage.

On being different: My earliest memory as a child is being in a crib with monitors everywhere, going to preschool and then coming home and having my mom talk to me about having surgery. Having surgery is second nature to me. When I was 6 years old I slept with a pulse oximetry machine and leads on my chest and I had a CPAP mask. I thought other kids dealt with that, too; I thought it was normal. I started to care when I was about 8 or 9. I started to understand better that I was different; I realized that I was the only kid with a plastic tube in her throat.

On the future: I have a dream that when I grow up I will start a foundation for kids who are in the special education system with learning disabilities and who people underestimate. I am what you call "doubly gifted." I have high test scores academically, but I have a hard time showing it on paper. Some teachers talk down to me and I have had trouble my whole life with being underestimated. I want to go around and tell kids that just because they are in special education does not mean that they do not have potential and that they are not smart. I want to let people know that nobody is disabled. People have unique challenges. There is no such thing as a disability and I want to make more people aware of that.

Kirsten Morrise is a student at Utah State University and is working on a children's book entitled A Lot Like You.

found out the hard way that just because you have one thing wrong doesn't mean that you won't have something else as well.

When Kirsten was 3 years old her seizures started getting worse. Kirsten's regular pediatrician was out of town, so I took her to see the pediatrician's colleague, who did not find anything significant. One grand mal seizure and three emergency room visits later, Kirsten was finally admitted to the hospital. Throughout this experience I was treated with great condescension, both by the residents in the hospital and by our pediatrician's colleague, who believed I simply was in denial about what he saw as the natural downward progress of Kirsten's condition. Even in the hospital they did not really do anything until Kirsten's neurologist happened by and told the residents that what was happening was not normal for her. They ordered a CT scan and a spinal tap. But the CT machine was broken and we had to wait for both until it got fixed later in the day.

For 3 days Kirsten had not had anything to drink, but nobody seemed to care that she was dehydrated. I could not seem to get people to hear me—I felt like I was in some kind of a horror nightmare. Eventually, they did the CT scan and the resident came in and said, "Well, the scan was clear. I am sure there is nothing there. We will probably send her home in the morning." About midnight the resident came running into the room with the results of the spinal tap. Kirsten had meningitis. She had something like 100 times the number of inflammatory cells in her spinal fluid that she should have had. They called in the infectious disease doctors and had to start an IV right away. They had to do to a cut-down to expose the vein after nine tries because it is really hard to start an IV on a dehydrated person. It was just a mess all the way around.

Before this happened, Kirsten could dress herself and was on her way to being potty trained at age 3. Afterward, she lost those skills and did not regain them until her second tracheotomy at the age of 8, when she picked up all her developmental loss. And again, a lot of people just kind of ran for the hills. They did not want to

> **Box 20-2 Running a Patient and Family Advisory Council: An Interview with Lisa Morrise**
>
> I began working with the children's medical center when I was asked to serve on their patient and family advisory council. I was intrigued because I saw great things happening at our children's hospital, but I also felt that I could not be the only person who encountered problems on a regular basis.
>
> I have a background in service-oriented organizations, so I had an idea about what an organization should look like. I was hired to help the council move from an advice and consent group—where the hospital would come to us and say, "We are going to do this; what do you think?"—to a structured group that has significantly altered the culture of our facility. We have patient advisors on hospital committees and we work on facility design and policies and procedures that have changed the way the hospital interacts with patients. We try to create an atmosphere in which patients feel welcomed and loved even when they are sick or in pain or need a procedure.
>
> One of the things that is central to my philosophy is building collaborative relations between providers and families. Our council includes social workers, child life nurses, and physicians, as well as administrators and families. Getting all these people on the same page doesn't just happen magically; it takes a coordinated effort. We are the same; we are all people, and we try to build relationships among the staff and families. We start every meeting checking in with a little reflection, and we share stories that are inspiring or motivational. We try to create a sense of camaraderie and a strong culture. It takes about a year for a new member to really get into the culture of the patient and family advisory council. It has been very meaningful for our family members to see how concerned and caring the staff are and how much they are seeking quality and process improvement.
>
> Lisa Morrise is a healthcare consultant and former manager of patient and family advisory councils in Salt Lake City, Utah.

apologize or say they were sorry. This was a very difficult experience for us. I was working at the time as a part-time manager for a radio network and I had to quit. That was the last job I had in my profession in my town. Since then people have said to me, "When Kirsten is better, come back and see us for a job," but she has never been totally better. I could not guarantee that I would not have to leave work for Kirsten's health-related issues, so that is what led me to work in the healthcare profession instead. **Box 20-2** presents an interview with Lisa Morrise and her involvement in running a patient and family advisory council.

Case Discussion

The healthcare exposure of the Morrises has spanned many years, yet many of the issues that have arisen over that time have been remarkably similar. Lisa Morrise describes two instances of delayed diagnosis that she believes had a profound effect on her daughter's life: the failure to recognize Kirsten's hypoxia for the first 2 hours of her life and the prolonged misinterpretation of Kirsten's symptoms of meningitis when she was 3 years old. In both cases, the mistakes seem to have arisen from healthcare professionals misreading the significance of her symptoms while downplaying the concerns of her mother. Another theme is the apparent unwillingness of Kirsten's caregivers to disclose and apologize for these two incidents. A significant oversight, in Lisa Morrise's opinion, was the failure to detect Kirsten's birth defect prenatally so that the obstetric team could be prepared for her special needs at delivery. Mrs. Morrise believes that more attention should have been paid to prenatal signs that Kirsten was affected by Pierre Robin sequence and that obstetric staff should routinely be trained on special circumstances in neonatal resuscitation, including Pierre Robin sequence. In her professional role in patient engagement and healthcare policy, she has also emphasized the importance of patient–provider collaboration to achieve the best results in health care.

Questions

1. What cognitive biases do you think might have contributed to the errors in Kirsten's care? What did they have in common? What does this say about the difficulties of diagnosis in patients with complex conditions?

2. Lisa Morrise mentions her shock at finding out that the hospital had been using her daughter's case as a training example for 16 years without ever telling the family that errors had occurred in Kirsten's treatment. Do you think the family should have been told about the errors that occurred at Kirsten's birth? Should a family be told if their loved one's events are being used for teaching? What practical and emotional effects do you think this lack of disclosure might have had on the family?

3. Do you think disclosure of adverse events is effectively done now? How do you think it could best be carried out?

4. Lisa Morrise is a highly educated and assertive family member. Even so, she felt that her concerns were not respected at several points in Kirsten's medical care. What are potential barriers to patient–provider collaboration, and how do you think those barriers could be overcome? What do you think is the best role for patient advisory councils?

5. Which of the core competencies for health professions do you think are most relevant for this case? Why?

References

American Heart Association in collaboration with the International Liaison Committee on Resuscitation. (2000). Guidelines 2000 for cardiopulmonary resuscitation and emergency cardiovascular care. Part 11: Neonatal resuscitation. *Circulation, 102*(Suppl 8), I343–I357.

Breugem, C. C., & Mink Van Der Molen, A. B. (2009). What is 'Pierre Robin sequence'? *Journal of Plastic, Reconstructive, and Aesthetic Surgery, 62*(12), 1555–1558.

Hsieh, Y. Y., Chang, C. C., Tsai, H. D., Yang, T. C., Lee, C. C., & Tsai, C. H. (1999). The prenatal diagnosis of Pierre-Robin sequence. *Prenatal Diagnosis, 19*(6), 567–569.

Shinghal, T., & Tewfik, T. (2008). Pierre Robin sequence: A common presentation. *Canadian Journal of CME*, September 8, 49–52.

Interprofessional Collaboration

Healthcare professionals must demonstrate the ability to engage in an interprofessional team in a manner that optimizes safe, effective patient- and population-centered care. Specific competencies within the Interprofessional Collaboration domain are to:

- Work with other health professionals to establish and maintain a climate of mutual respect, dignity, diversity, ethical integrity, and trust.

- Use the knowledge of one's own role and the roles of other health professionals to appropriately assess and address the healthcare needs of the patients and populations served.

- Communicate with other health professionals in a responsive and responsible manner that supports the maintenance of health and the treatment of disease in individual patients and populations.

- Participate in different team roles to establish, develop, and continuously enhance interprofessional teams to provide patient- and population-centered care that is safe, timely, efficient, effective, and equitable.

Case 21, "Failure to Rescue," is the story of DJ Sterner. DJ's wife, Karen Sterner, and his mother, Linda Ward, tell the story of DJ's battle with cancer. DJ was diagnosed with thyroid lymphoma at the age of 47. He was successfully treated and the cancer was in remission, but he later discovered that he had developed a second cancer, acute myeloid leukemia, likely caused by the chemotherapy he had received. DJ was admitted to the hospital for more chemotherapy and died while in the hospital from *Clostridium perfringens*, a typically food-borne infection to which immunosuppressed individuals like chemotherapy patients can be vulnerable.

In Case 22, "Unmonitored: A Postsurgical Narcotic Overdose in the Hospital," Laura Townsend recalls the events that led to her mother's postoperative death in San Antonio, Texas. Louise Batz was 65 years old when she underwent knee replacement surgery. The surgery was apparently successful, but on the first night after surgery Louise was given a combination of Demerol, Vistaril, and morphine. She went into respiratory depression and suffered an anoxic brain injury. Louise died in the hospital 11 days later.

Case 23, "The Voice That Is Missing: A Mother's Journey in Patient Safety Advocacy," is a discussion by Ilene Corina about the circumstances that led to the death of her 2-year-old son Michael following what should have been a routine tonsillectomy. Ilene talks about the ways in which the lessons from Michael's death helped facilitate her interaction with the healthcare establishment when Michael's younger brother was born prematurely, and she reflects on how both of these experiences helped shape her subsequent pathway as a patient advocate devoted to community-based action in patient safety.

The final case in this section, Case 24, "When Healing Harms: Recovering from a Multisystem Traumatic Injury," is the story of New Zealand resident Kathy Torpie, who writes about her experience as a patient with multiple traumatic injuries from a severe, near-fatal automobile accident. In the 17 years following the accident, Kathy underwent dozens of surgeries, some of which were necessitated by earlier errors and omissions in her medical treatment. Kathy focuses on several episodes from her healthcare journey to highlight ways to alleviate the system's issues that she sees as leading to unnecessary suffering for patients and overuse of resources for the healthcare system.

The cases presented in this section are complex and include elements of multiple interrelated competencies. As you read the cases, it is helpful to think about the other competencies that are relevant. (Refer to the full list of competencies in the appendix.)

Failure to Rescue

The Story of DJ Sterner (United States)

Karen Sterner and Linda Ward

Editors' Note

DJ Sterner was a friendly, gregarious truck driver. Together with his wife Karen, he traveled all 48 of the mainland United States in his 18-wheel tractor-trailer. A big man with an open face, DJ was active, generous, and loved to help others. He helped neighbors with car repairs, did chores for those who were incapacitated, and looked after his relatives when they were ill. While he was on the road, he was involved in a pen pal program for school-children called the "trucker buddy" program. He and Karen would visit classrooms, talk to the children about trucking, and give them a tour of his Freightliner Century Class truck and its 53-foot trailer. They would send the children postcards from their travels, trying to incorporate lessons in geography with real-life stories of what a long-haul trucker really does.

DJ was diagnosed at the age of 47 with thyroid lymphoma, a rare cancer. After 6 months of chemotherapy, he was told the cancer was in remission. About a year later, he was informed that he had developed a second cancer, acute myeloid leukemia, known to be a potential side effect of the chemotherapy he had received. DJ was admitted to the hospital for more chemotherapy, developed an infection, and died. DJ's wife Karen and his mother Linda Ward tell the story of DJ's odyssey through the medical system and his last days in the hospital.

LEARNING OBJECTIVES

After completing this case study, you will be able to:

1. Explore the role of rapid response teams and other mechanisms for responding to patients in crisis.

2. Discuss elements of a strategy to include patients and family members in care decisions.

3. Discuss barriers to an effective informed consent process.

4. Analyze the issue of bias in treatment of patients with a terminal illness.

A Cancer Diagnosis . . . Twice

My husband DJ was diagnosed in June 2009 with an enlarged thyroid gland that was pressing on his trachea and esophagus. We made a trip to the emergency room and found out that he had thyroid lymphoma, a very rare cancer. His endocrinologist told us that there are only two cases per 1 million people in the United States for this particular type of cancer, but he also said that this rare cancer responds very well to chemotherapy.

DJ started chemotherapy just a couple of weeks after his diagnosis and continued therapy from June through November 2009. His treating oncologist never gave us any specific numbers in regard to remission or cure, but I found an article that said that 85% of patients are cured with CHOP, a chemotherapy regimen consisting of cyclophosphamide, doxorubicin, vincristine, and prednisone (Cabanellas, 2012). DJ received this regimen plus an additional biotherapy agent.

By the end of his chemotherapy regimen in November, DJ was considered to be in remission. He had had a CT scan after the first four rounds of chemo, which was halfway through his treatment regimen. He had another scan a couple of weeks after he finished his chemo sessions, and another one 3 months after the treatment ended. We were told that all the CT scans were clear and that there were no signs of cancer. His chemotherapy port was removed in May 2010.

A few months later, in August 2010, we noticed that DJ's face was starting to get very pale. He seemed fatigued and his lymph nodes were swollen. His oncologist decided that he needed to have a lymph node biopsy. Approximately a week after the biopsy, on September 10, 2010, he was diagnosed with acute myeloid leukemia.

One of the hospital oncologists later looked at DJ's medical records and said to us, "The chemo caused this." We were stunned to hear this news, as we had never been told about the possibility of this severe side effect. After the first four rounds of chemotherapy, DJ's follow-up CT scan had showed no more cancer. It was never explained to us why we continued with the chemotherapy after that. Was he really gaining any benefit or was he just basically increasing his chances of side effects? If DJ had known that acute myeloid leukemia was a possible side effect of the chemotherapy, I think he might have discontinued the chemotherapy, received lower doses, or possibly continued with biotherapy treatment only.

There was a lot of evidence that the chemotherapy caused DJ's acute myeloid leukemia. His bone marrow biopsy was negative at the time of his thyroid lymphoma diagnosis, so we know he did not have leukemia before he began the treatment. A leukemia expert at Tulane University later confirmed that it was therapy-related leukemia, and DJ's cytogenetic testing revealed that he had a common gene translocation for therapy-related leukemia (De Braekeleer et al., 2005). The forensic pathologist even alluded to the cause of the illness in the autopsy report. He described therapy-related leukemia and listed the two types of chemotherapy agents (doxorubicin and cyclophosphamide) known to cause acute leukemia. DJ had received both these chemo agents as part of the CHOP chemotherapy regimen.

DJ's Hospital Stay

When DJ received the diagnosis of acute myeloid leukemia, his primary doctor said that he had a poor prognosis. Later, one of his oncologists told us that chemotherapy-related leukemia is hard to treat and that DJ would probably need to have a bone marrow transplant within 6–9 months.

The doctors wanted to act fast. DJ received his diagnosis of acute myeloid leukemia on a Friday. The next day, Saturday, September 11, 2010, he was admitted to the hospital, because they wanted to start chemotherapy on Monday. But then on Monday, they performed a bone marrow biopsy. They had done an outside consultation for his lymph node biopsy and wanted to be sure they had correctly identified the leukemia. On Tuesday, the oncologist came to the hospital and confirmed that DJ had acute myeloid leukemia. The following day, Wednesday, he actually started chemotherapy.

We knew he was going to be in the hospital for a long time because they planned an intense 24/7 chemotherapy treatment instead of outpatient chemo treatments. DJ was doing well; he was in good spirits. We were totally blown away with the courage that he showed during this whole thing. He went out of his way to put everybody else at ease. He joked, he laughed. You would not believe that he had poor prognosis cancer by the way he acted.

On Saturday, September 18, a week after he was admitted, DJ started vomiting in the morning after breakfast. He vomited three times between 10:00 a.m. and noon. He was complaining of cramps in his lower rib cage area, and it kept getting worse. Even with two morphine shots his pain did not subside. He began to breathe rapidly, and this got worse throughout the day. He also felt like he was constipated. He went back and forth to the toilet at least 20 times, trying to get relief but to no avail. In addition, he was fidgeting every few seconds in his bed due to his severe discomfort. In desperation, he called his parents to bring his TENS pain management machine[1] from home, but his pain was unrelenting and excruciating.

The nurse told us that DJ was just having anxiety, but we thought it was something more serious. His nurse gave him Ativan for anxiety, but when we asked what it was the nurse responded with a technical term, as if he was trying to hide what he was giving him. The nurse knew we did not agree with his assessment.

The attending physician came in around 2:00 p.m. and ordered an abdominal x-ray. A few minutes after the x-ray was taken, we were told that it was normal. Another doctor, the on-call oncologist, came in just after 2:00 p.m. He asked DJ if he was in pain. DJ responded that he was. The doctor pressed on different parts of his stomach area and asked if he felt pain. DJ kept saying, "Yes!" His face clearly indicated that he was in serious pain. The doctor made a startled face and walked out of the room. He did not order any test or give us any indication of what was really going on. It felt as though he was dismissing DJ. We never saw this doctor again.

DJ was in agony all afternoon. He breathing was very shallow, just a pant. We did not realize at the time how serious this was or we would have been out in the hall screaming for help. If a doctor had walked in, they would have realized how serious DJ's condition was.

Around 3:00 p.m. the nurses began trying to page the doctor to tell him that something was wrong. DJ's pain was not going away, his cramping was getting worse, and his breathing was getting worse. The nurse came in and told us she had spoken to the doctor and that he had told her he was coming, but an hour went by and still he was not there.

The nurses made seven calls approximately half an hour to an hour apart up until 7:00 that evening. The doctors never responded. Every time they were called, there was nothing. At one time a doctor who was called assumed that the other doctor had already been to DJ's room. So there was miscommunication, but the miscommunication was never corrected.

---

[1] A TENS, or transcutaneous electrical nerve stimulation, unit is a portable unit that uses electrical current transmitted through electrodes on the skin to try to relieve nerve pain. DJ had a TENS unit that he had used for pain from an old back injury and subsequent spinal fusion surgery.

The two doctors who did not respond were both residents. One was an intern and one was a second- or third-year resident. The attending physician was not called.

DJ finally threw his hands up in the air and said, "That's it. I want sedation." I was very surprised because it was totally out of character for him to be complaining of pain. He told us he was scared. He even said to his nurse, "Please make it stop." We knew something was very serious for him to be talking this way. I actually had a confrontation with one of the nurses out in the hallway because of this.

His nurse checked his respiration around 6:30 p.m. and it was around 20. Then they checked it again around shift change at 7:00 p.m. and it was closer to 30. His blood pressure was really low and his blood oxygen level was 43%. At that point his nurse paged another doctor overhead.

By the time the doctor arrived, DJ had passed out. The nurse called a code, and it took only *2 minutes* for the resuscitation response team to get to the room. When the respiratory therapist walked through the door she said to the assistant next to her, "I knew he was in trouble before I got through the door."

The assistant replied, "Why didn't they call us sooner?"

The critical response team gave DJ oxygen and he was transferred to the intensive care unit. After we got there, the intensive care doctor took us out into the hallway and told us that DJ had an infection in his abdomen, that he had gone into septic shock, and that he had lactic acidosis.

DJ rapidly deteriorated from there. Throughout the night his abdomen became more and more distended. He looked as though he was 9 months pregnant. His blood pressure continued to drop, even though he was given medications. They could not find a pulse.

Finally, the next morning he went into cardiac arrest. They were able to revive him, but his blood pressure continued to drop and finally he died. It was September 19, 2010. His symptoms had begun 24 hours earlier.

Conclusion

DJ's primary doctor at the hospital didn't really quite understand what had happened. He said it was not normal for someone to deteriorate rapidly like that. The doctor had questions himself, so he ordered an autopsy, and I consented to the autopsy. The autopsy report showed that the direct cause of death was acute hemorrhagic necrotizing enterocolitis. The report said that there were no signs of residual or recurrent lymphoma of the thyroid. Both the duodenum (the first part of the small intestine) and the sigmoid colon (the last part of the large intestine) had hemorrhaged or broken down. The report named the pathogen: *Clostridium perfringens* bacteria.

We asked the primary doctor how DJ could have contracted that kind of infection in the hospital. He gave us a very vague answer. We ended up doing our own research and found out from the FDA's website that this infection is commonly associated with food poisoning. *C. perfringens* can grow on cooked food that has been left too long at room temperature, and it is often implicated in food poisoning outbreaks in large institutions like hospitals, where food may be kept at room temperature while waiting to be served (Al-Khaldi, 2012).

Case Discussion

C. perfringens food poisoning is usually caused by a strain of *C. perfringens* called type A and normally consists of about 1 day of comparatively mild cramps and diarrhea. A very severe form of the illness, thought to be extremely rare, is caused by type C strains of *C. perfringens* and leads to necrotizing enteritis (intestinal tissue death). A similar severe syndrome called neutropenic enterocolitis occurs in leukemia patients, cancer patients undergoing chemotherapy, and other immunosuppressed individuals, and is often associated with a related pathogen, *C. septicum*. Case reports over the past decade, however, have documented fast-moving, often fatal, cases of necrotizing enterocolitis associated with the type A strain of *C. perfringens*. The majority of these illnesses appear to be foodborne (Bos et al., 2005; Minisini et al., 2011; Sobel et al., 2005). These reports have much in common with what happened to DJ.

The fact that DJ died in severe pain has continued to haunt his family. His wife and mother consider that their concerns were dismissed and feel strongly that the option of a patient-activated rapid response team should have been made available to patients in this hospital. They also thought that the significance of what happened to DJ was dismissed after death. When his doctor discussed the autopsy report with the family, he said, "Since he had leukemia, his prognosis was poor." The family felt that DJ did not get the care he needed in the hospital, and that even in the postmortem analysis his final illness and the lessons that might come from it were treated as unimportant because he had a serious cancer diagnosis.

The family filed a complaint with the state health department. The complaint was substantiated, and the hospital was cited for four deficiencies of care. One of the major deficiencies was that DJ's resident physicians did not respond between the hours of 3:00 and 8:00 p.m., even though the record shows that they were paged seven times. They were cited for not responding to the nurses' pages in a timely manner. The hospital was also cited for failing to notify the state health department about DJ's *C. perfringens* infection, a foodborne illness that is required to be reported to the authorities. They also failed to report the unexpected death of a patient from a condition not directly related to his hospitalization, another state requirement. Finally, they were cited for not authenticating verbal physician orders. Several orders that were executed during DJ's stay were not authenticated until a month later.

Questions

1. DJ Sterner began to decline on a Saturday and he died on a Sunday. Discuss the problem of low nurse and physician staffing on nights and weekends and how it might affect patient care. What can the individual healthcare professional do to help improve this situation?

2. An unattended decline like that suffered by DJ is considered "failure to rescue." This results from bedside staff either failing to recognize or failing to respond to the fact that the patient is deteriorating. What do you think are the barriers to getting immediate help for a patient in trouble? How can these barriers be overcome? What could DJ's nurses have done when they did not get a response to their pages?

3. Research the effectiveness of rapid response teams and other mechanisms for responding to patients in crisis. Why do you think that DJ's nurses did not call the rapid response team that was available? Explore patient-activated rapid response teams.

4. Regulatory authorities sanctioned DJ's hospital for failure to report two incidents relating to his case: a reportable illness and an unexpected death. Studies show that adverse events in hospitals are severely underreported. Why do you think this is? What is the importance of reporting adverse events, and how can reporting be increased?

5. DJ's family felt that they had been misled when they were not told that his chemotherapy could lead to secondary cancers. They believed they should have been given more choices in DJ's treatment. What do you think is the best way to involve patients in decisions about their treatment? What dilemma does this present for the healthcare professional who feels strongly that one course of treatment is preferable over another?

6. DJ's family also felt that his agonizing death was dismissed as insignificant because of his terminal cancer diagnosis. This

perception caused them much emotional anguish because they felt that DJ's suffering and his value as a person were disregarded. How could his doctors have handled this differently?

7. Leukemia patients and other immunocompromised individuals are especially vulnerable to foodborne illness and other infections. Research what precautions can be taken to try to avert infection in immunocompromised patients. What foods should be avoided?

8. Which of the core competencies for health professions are most relevant for this case? Why?

References

Al-Khaldi, S. (2012). *Clostridium perfringens.* In: K. A. Lampel, S. Al-Khaldi, & S. M. Cahill (Eds.), *Bad bug book: Foodborne pathogenic microorganisms and natural toxins handbook* (2nd ed.). Washington, D.C.: United States Food and Drug Administration.

Bos, J., Smithee, L., McClane, B., Distefano, R. F., Uzal, F., Songer, J. G., ... Crutcher, J. M. (2005). Fatal necrotizing colitis following a food-borne outbreak of enterotoxigenic *Clostridium perfringens* type A infection. *Clinical Infectious Diseases, 40*(10), e78–e83.

Cabanillas, F. (2012). Thyroid lymphoma. Medscape Reference. Available at: http://emedicine.medscape.com/article/281983.

De Braekeleer, M., Morel, F., Le Bris, M. J., Herry, A., & Douet-Guilbert, N. (2005). The MLL gene and translocations involving chromosomal band 11q23 in acute leukemia. *Anticancer Research, 25*(3B), 1931–1944.

Minisini, A. M., Menis, J., Follador, A., Avellini, C., & Fasola, G. (2011). Fulminating septic shock from *Clostridium perfringens* in an early breast cancer patient with severe myalgia after docetaxel treatment. *Clinics and Practices, 1*(2), e32.

Sobel, J., Mixter, C. G., Kolhe, P., Gupta, A., Guarner, J., Zaki, S., ... MacDonald, C. (2005). Necrotizing enterocolitis associated with *Clostridium perfringens* type A in previously healthy North American adults. *Journal of the American College of Surgeons, 201*(1), 48–56.

Unmonitored: A Postsurgical Narcotic Overdose in the Hospital

The Story of Louise Batz
(United States)

Laura Townsend

Editors' Note

Laura Townsend, daughter of Louise Batz, recalls the events that led to her mother's death from a narcotic overdose after surgery. She talks about her family's discovery of the facts surrounding her mother's death and the family's subsequent efforts to improve patient safety and the monitoring of postsurgical patients in hospitals.

LEARNING OBJECTIVES

After completing this case study, you will be able to:

1. Give examples of the vulnerability of surgical patients throughout the perisurgical continuum and discuss how best to keep them safe.
2. Summarize the risks of narcotic and sedative medications, which are responsible for a high number of adverse medication events.
3. Outline communication strategies among doctor, nurse, and family that can help prevent adverse events.
4. Discuss ways in which patient and family education can improve patient care and how it can best be achieved.

A Knee Replacement

I remember it like it was yesterday, that is how fresh it all stays in your mind. On the day after Easter, 2009, my mother was getting ready to have routine knee replacement surgery. I had come to stay with her before her surgery and we were watching television. My mother was 65 years old, and she was a very thorough person. She had all her paperwork for the hospital, and she was reading through everything while we watched TV. She was calm and ready to have the surgery. She had timed it carefully so she would have time to heal and be ready for the arrival of her fourth grandchild.

This surgery wasn't something that she had jumped into. She had tried for a couple of years to find medical options, but she had severe arthritis that made it painful to walk. She finally concluded that knee surgery was the only solution. She had seen a physical therapist and had been receiving steroid shots from the surgeon who would do the knee replacement. She always commented on how impressed she was with him and how it never hurt when he gave her the steroid shots.

There was another knee surgeon whom she had known for years, but he was older and people said his shots hurt. So she chose this new one. My mom also chose this doctor because the hospital where he did surgery was close to the house. My father had recently had heart bypass surgery, so my mother wanted it to be a close drive for him to visit her in the hospital. I met the doctor, too, and I liked him. I still think he is a good surgeon.

The morning of surgery my father, my aunt, and I went with my mom into the preoperative area. That was where my aunt caught the first big mistake. They were about to operate on two knees instead of just one! Honestly, if my aunt hadn't been there my mom would have probably come back with two repaired knees instead of the one she went in for.

The surgery lasted about an hour and a half. The surgeon came out and told us she had a beautiful new knee, that the surgery had gone well, and that she would be in the hospital for 3 days. When I asked, he told me he would not be back that day to see her. That should have been a red flag to me. It was very different from our past experiences, when doctors would always come back and check on us. This was partly because they knew us, as we have five doctors in our family: my grandfather, my brother, my uncle, my sister-in-law, and my aunt. Other doctors were usually available to us as friends and colleagues.

Mom went to her room on the orthopedic unit. She did great all day. They put a contraption on her knee that completely immobilized her so there was absolutely no way for her to get out of bed. She was given a patient-controlled analgesia (PCA) pump, and the nurse pushed the button to give her a bolus infusion of 2 mg of morphine. This worked well to control her pain. Then at 6:00 p.m. they gave her some creamy soup that made her feel nauseated, so they gave her an antihistamine, Vistaril, which was supposed to help with nausea but also made her sleepy. I left soon thereafter.

After dinner, I came back with my little girl, Ella, who was 4 years old. My mother and my daughter had a special relationship. Mom would take care of Ella at least once or twice a week. I am so glad I brought her because, although none of us knew it, this was the last time Ella would see her grandmother.

I took Ella home and came back around 9:30 p.m. My dad and I sat with the nurse and went over my mom's medications for the night. At midnight Mom was scheduled to get Vistaril, Demerol, and more morphine from the PCA pump. We told the nurse that Mom was not nauseated anymore so she really didn't need the Vistaril and she didn't need the Demerol either. We were concerned that with three sedating drugs she might be overmedicated. My mother wasn't a person who liked to take a lot of medications. The most she ever took at home was ibuprofen. And she wasn't in much pain; she told them that she was fine and that she couldn't really feel the pain.

The nurse asked us to go home for the night because Mom needed to rest. So I gave Mom a kiss and told her how proud I was of her, and my dad and I left. I never imagined that would be the last time I would get to talk to her or tell her goodnight and that I loved her. I will forever wish that I had not listened to that nurse. I will always wish that I had stayed with her.

Trouble Breathing

My dad and I were in such relief at this point. We were so happy that things were going well. But he was not excited about going home without Mom. They were always together. I think that during their 50 years of marriage my parents had maybe spent 2 weeks apart from each other.

Dad and I sat up and visited until around midnight and then we decided to go to bed. At about 3:15 a.m. my dad received a phone call that my mother was having trouble breathing. We raced to the hospital. As I ran down the hall to her room, I saw a security guard outside her door. My chest tightened and my heart sank. Something was very wrong. Why would they have a security guard outside her door? I raced into her room, and at that moment I felt a pain that I have never experienced in my life. I thought my mom was already dead. She was so white and lying so still on the bed. The nurse was pumping oxygen into her. She could not breathe on her own. Now I knew why they had a security guard. I think they were afraid of how we might react.

At that point I just began to get angry. The nurse had given her Demerol, Vistaril, and morphine at midnight and then had never gone back to check on her. My mom had gone into respiratory depression and suffered an anoxic brain injury.

I started yelling and screaming, and it took every ounce of me not to start throwing things at them. How could this have happened to my sweet wonderful mother? It is so hard to describe the emotions that I felt at that moment. It was like a thousand knives going straight through my body.

I called one of my mother's dear friends who was an emergency medicine doctor at the hospital. He was there within 15 minutes and helped to get the team together. I will be forever grateful to that doctor. They put my mom in hypothermia with ice to try to protect her brain and reduce the brain swelling from the anoxic injury. They tried desperately to save my mom so that our family and friends might have the opportunity to be with her one last time.

My mother was in the hospital for 11 days before she died. During that time family and friends showered us with love and support. It was truly amazing and a tribute to how much people loved her. I sat with her during the days and nights. It was the first time I had ever taken care of Mom. When I was growing up, she was never sick. I can only remember one or two times in my entire life when Mom was too sick to take care of us, and even then it was only for a day. I held her hand, massaged her feet, and put ice packs on her forehead when her fever would get high. I just wanted to try to take care of her the way she had always cared for me.

I kept hoping for a miracle. But the damage to Mom's brain was too massive, and 8 days later we were told that she would never recover. On April 26, 2009, we made the decision to take her off the breathing machine. I held her hand and stroked her head while she was fighting, unconsciously, to breathe. I begged her to stop struggling. I told her that it was time for her to go to heaven and that she could take care of us from up there. My Aunt Joanne was holding her other hand and telling her the same thing. My brother paced the hall. He couldn't bear to see her struggling to breathe. My brother's wife, Ginger, sat at the corner of the bed, her head down, crying. My husband Michael stood behind me rubbing my shoulders. He never left my side. My dad was sitting in the chair next to her in shock. His eyes were glazed over. He was a man with a broken heart.

I looked up at the monitors. Her oxygen saturation finally read zero and the heart monitor had flatlined. My mom had passed away. I went into the hallway and sat on the floor, crying. I was terrified because I couldn't feel my mom anymore. We always had a very special connection, and for the first time I couldn't feel it. I was so scared. But I was blessed by her love for 35 years. I will always have those memories and moments in my heart.

How Could This Happen?

During those long 11 days in the hospital I had a lot of time to think and I wondered if we were the only people who had ever gone through this, or if this happened on a regular basis. How could this happen, even in a family of five doctors? I started doing some research and quickly realized what a huge problem patient safety is in this country. The few hours each day that I was not at the hospital with my mom, I kept diving into research and learning as much as I could about patient safety. I had no idea so many people died each year from preventable medical mistakes. The ironic thing is that neither did my family members who are doctors. They had thought it was very rare.

After meeting with the hospital doctors and nurses, we felt there were three things that really went wrong for my mom that day. First of all, there was a lack of teamwork, which underpinned all the errors that happened throughout that day.

Second, there was a lack of knowledge on the part of the family and the patient. We asked a thousand questions that day, but we didn't get lucky and ask the right ones. I didn't know the right questions to ask to help my mom get through this experience.

The third thing was the lack of technology. There were no monitors on my mom to measure her breathing and heart rate. She was not being monitored at all. Since mom's death I have researched PCA pump safety and have learned that patients need to be continuously monitored when they are on PCA pumps because of the risk of respiratory depression from the PCA narcotics.

I can't sit and point fingers at a specific doctor or nurse. It was the system that was in place that let my mom down. My mom only had one chance, and she lost it because people weren't working together as a team. I feel that the best we can do is to move forward and help other people so that this doesn't happen again.

Conclusion

I vowed that my mom's legacy wasn't going to be on that bed dying. That wasn't her life. She was such a joyful, hopeful person; that wasn't going to be her legacy. So the night my mother died I began writing the mission for what became the Louise H. Batz Patient Safety Foundation. We started the foundation basically right after the memorial service. We worked very hard as a family, and we brought the community together to work on the foundation.

We began to figure out how we could make a better experience for other families and help them not go through the pain that we had gone through. We developed the Batz patient guide (Townsend & Armbruster, 2010), which takes you through the whole process of hospitalization from before surgery, during surgery, all the way to discharge. We worked with doctors, nurses, hospital administrators, and patient safety leaders together as a team, because we felt that if patients and families are not part of the team there will always be errors.

My mom always turned every stone over and did everything she could to help others. She had that "never give up" attitude. We try to do the same thing with her foundation. We have implemented the guide in hospitals; we have developed a mobile application; we have created guides for special populations like pediatrics. We feel that our work takes this tragedy and makes it hopeful. Our hope is to help nurses and doctors by becoming part of the team.

Case Discussion

Louise Batz entered the hospital for a knee replacement and suffered irreversible brain injury due to narcotic overdose less than 24 hours later. The shock her family felt was compounded by the fact that Mrs. Batz's postsurgical pain was not severe. Her husband and daughter had reviewed her medications in detail with her bedside nurse and were confident in their belief that the nurse had agreed not to give two of the three drugs. They were upset not only that the nurse gave the medications in spite of their verbal understanding, but that the nurse then failed to check to make sure the patient was tolerating the combination of sedatives and narcotics.

Once they had a chance to research the topic, the family was also disturbed to realize that Mrs. Batz had received no continuous electronic monitoring. Although it is still far from universal, monitoring with technologies like pulse oximetry is considered best practice for postsurgical patients on narcotic pain medications (Weinger & Lee, 2011). Monitoring is particularly important for patients on PCA pumps, a powerful technology that hospital systems are not always mature enough to handle safely. Adverse medication events involving PCA pumps can stem from healthcare professionals' failure to appreciate the impact of the continuous background drip of patient-controlled analgesia, which can allow additional drugs to push the patient over the edge and cause respiratory depression. Continuous monitoring can lessen the likelihood of such an event.

Louise Batz's family attributed her death not only to lack of monitoring, but also to lack of teamwork among the various professionals involved in her care. They felt that communication was poor between nurse and doctor and that their wishes as family members were disregarded, effectively keeping them from being part of the team. They were particularly concerned that the surgeon whose orders were so uncritically followed seemed to have little direct personal involvement in his patient's postsurgical care.

Finally, Mrs. Batz's family blamed her death on the family's own lack of knowledge, including that of Louise Batz herself. Mrs. Batz had chosen her surgeon and made her decision on where to have the surgery on the basis of reasons that were not trivial, but that were not medically informed or concerned with potential variations in the quality of care. Once in the hospital, Mrs. Batz's daughter Laura felt that she had not known the questions to ask or how to navigate the system to prevent her mother's medication error. Together with her family and other collaborators, she has attempted to bridge that gap by creating a series of patient guides intended to help patients and families play a more effective part in their own care.

Questions

1. What are the best practices for patient-controlled analgesia? How were they violated in this case?

2. Research the different kinds of monitoring that are available for patients taking narcotics in hospitals when being cared for with PCA pumps. Which do you think is most effective? Which is most practical?

3. Discuss the ways in which communication breakdown might have contributed to Mrs. Batz's death.

4. What do you think of the idea that patients and families need to be responsible for maintaining vigilance over the patient's well-being? Should this be considered a failure of the medical system or a sign of progress in making the patient and their family an integral part of the medical team?

5. How do you think that healthcare professionals can contribute to improving patient knowledge and making patients more involved and empowered?

6. Mrs. Batz's family had requested that she not receive more pain medication even though the doctor had ordered it. The nurse gave it to her anyway. What should a nurse do in the situation in which a family's wishes conflict with the doctor's orders?

7. Research which medications are responsible for the majority of adverse medication events. What is the risk profile for the narcotics and sedatives involved in Louise Batz's overdose? What patient factors should influence dosing?

8. Explore the field of human factors and how they influence the look, feel, and function of medical devices and infusion pumps like the one Louise Batz was on. Should patients and families have a basic knowledge of how medical devices and infusion pumps work and how they can malfunction?

9. Which of the core competencies for health professions are most relevant for this case? Why?

References

Townsend, L. B., & Armbruster, R. (Eds.). (2010). *The Batz guide for bedside advocacy*. San Antonio: Louise H. Batz Patient Safety Foundation. Available at: http://www.louisebatz.org.

Weinger, M. B., & Lee, L. A. for the Anesthesia Patient Safety Foundation. (2011). No patient shall be harmed by opioid-induced respiratory depression: Proceedings of the Essential Monitoring Strategies to Detect Clinically Significant Drug-Induced Respiratory Depression in the Postoperative Period conference. *APSF Newsletter*, 26(2), 21–40.

The Voice That Is Missing: A Mother's Journey in Patient Safety Advocacy

The Story of Michael Corina (United States)

Julie K Johnson, Helen Haskell, and Paul Barach

Editors' Note

Michael Corina was almost 3 years old when he died from profuse hemorrhage following a tonsillectomy and adenoidectomy. In an interview with the editors, Michael's mother, Ilene Corina, discussed the events surrounding his death and reflected on how that experience influenced her interactions with the healthcare system when she later delivered a premature infant. Her personal journey inspired her to found PULSE NY, a leading patient advocacy organization. The following account is taken from an interview with Ilene Corina conducted on December 6, 2011.

LEARNING OBJECTIVES

After completing this case study, you will be able to:

1. Explain the value of shared decision making in helping patients and families assess the balance between the risk and benefit of a procedure.

2. Examine ways in which patient information on a doctor's background might affect patient care.

3. Relate strategies to promote patient and family participation in their own health care.

4. Assess the ways in which patient action in communities can help improve healthcare quality and safety.

A Smart Little Boy

My firstborn son, Michael, was the first grandchild in our family and was my only child at the time. Michael was a really smart little boy. We spent a lot of time in doctor's offices because of his chronic ear infections, and we had time on our hands in the waiting room. I always carried flash cards with me because cards, I learned, were fun, educational, and didn't take up much room. Michael knew the whole alphabet and all his numbers at a very early age and was reading by the time he was 2.

When Michael was almost 3 years old we decided that he needed his tonsils and adenoids removed and tubes put in his ears. I did everything I thought I was supposed to do. At that time, I interviewed doctors, and I chose the one I felt was the nicest doctor. I did not know how to check their backgrounds. I did not know how to choose a doctor, so I chose somebody who was really nice and had a young child like Michael.

The doctor discussed the risks of putting a child to sleep twice and said that it was better to do all the surgeries at once. We actually canceled the surgery twice because Michael was sick with another ear infection. So the doctor felt that we should do it all together so we would not have to put him under more than once. This did make sense to me. But everything in our discussion before the surgery was about the anesthesia and not about the surgery.

Michael had the tonsillectomy/adenoidectomy and had the tubes placed in his ears. He was sent home that night. The doctor gave us a number to call if there were any problems.

Blood on the Pillow

This was on a Tuesday. Two days later, on Thursday, my son woke up from a nap with blood on his pillow. I called the surgeon and told him that something was not right, that Michael had been bleeding from the mouth. So I brought him back to the surgeon, and the surgeon cauterized the spot where he saw bleeding.

The next day Michael was fine. But then, that Saturday, he started throwing up blood clots. I called the hospital and told them I needed to bring my son in. The hospital kept putting me on hold. I asked if I should call 911 and they told me no. After being placed on hold a few times I hung up the phone and brought him into the hospital.

In the emergency room they looked at Michael's throat and could not find where the bleeding was coming from. I didn't feel that they believed me about how heavy his bleeding was even though my shirt was covered in blood. I had held my son while he was throwing up to try to comfort him. The sweatshirt I was wearing was drenched in his blood, but it couldn't be seen because the fabric was dark blue and the blood had soaked into it. The only odd thing was that his temperature was very low. I was happy about a low temperature because he had always had fevers as an infant. I remember saying, "Thank God he doesn't have a fever; this is the first time he has not had a fever!" I found out much later that a very low temperature is one of the symptoms of going into shock. I did not know to ask about fever or what a low temperature meant.

Michael was calm at the time and the emergency room staff told me to go see his surgeon that afternoon. So I called but I could not reach the surgeon, and staff would not help me reach him. Instead, they said to see the pediatrician on call, so we saw a pediatrician instead. I brought him in to see the pediatrician that same afternoon; she looked in Michael's throat and said he was fine, not to worry about it, and to take him home.

We went home. Michael was acting okay. But the next day, Sunday, he had huge welts on his buttocks, and his penis and groin area were swollen.

That afternoon there was blood in his teeth. So that afternoon we went to a different emergency room. The doctor said he did not see where the bleeding was coming from, and he gave us a prescription for an ointment for the sores on his behind.

We got the prescription filled and placed the ointment on the sores. The next day, on Monday night, we went for the 1-week check-up with Michael's surgeon. I told the surgeon what had happened. The surgeon said, "It's a good thing they didn't call me, because I would have put him back into the hospital."

The surgeon checked my son and said that whatever they had done was fine. He told us to keep him on liquids for a few more days and he sent us home.

On Tuesday, I took Michael to the babysitter and went back to work. While I was at work I got a phone call from the babysitter, who said Michael was throwing up huge amounts of blood. I immediately called the doctor's office while the babysitter called 911.

When I got to the babysitter's house just 3 miles away, I grabbed my son and held him. He lay limp in my arms and didn't seem to know I was there. Then the paramedics took my son from my arms, and that was the last I ever saw of him.

I went to the hospital and sat in the emergency room with Michael's babysitter. The head of pediatrics kept coming in and telling us that "they were working on him." Then she came back and told us that "he had not survived."

The words made me cold, as if she were talking to someone else. I didn't cry. I just asked if we could donate any part of him. We donated his eyes. Nothing else could be preserved because they had done too much damage to his organs trying to save him.

He was filled with infection. I found out later that his blisters were infections and that he was hemorrhaging inside. He was swallowing the blood, and the large amount that he threw up was all in his stomach. The autopsy confirmed that there was blood in his stomach.

Reflections

The hardest part of going through that week was the fact that I was saying, "Something is not right" and trusting the healthcare providers when they told me everything was okay. Michael had every sign of being in shock, and nobody took my concerns seriously. In the emergency room, I felt that they didn't believe what I told them about the amount of blood he was throwing up and how severe it was. It was Saturday morning and the staff just did not want to hear it. They were too busy with other things.

If I had had a support system at that time to support me in insisting that something was not right I think the outcome could have been very different. I would have felt empowered to follow my instincts and say, "I am not leaving until somebody makes sure he is okay," because that is what I would do now. I think there were a lot of things that could have been done differently if I had known that people die from surgery, that people can die from medical treatment.

One of the things that has stayed with me forever is that I really liked the surgeon. I chose him because I liked him and trusted him, and that did not immediately change. So on top of the fact that my son had died I had to question my own judgment. Did I choose the wrong person to entrust my child to?

The surgeon did call and said he did not know what had happened and asked me if I had any questions for him. I asked if I could talk to him when I received the autopsy report. So we talked for just a matter of minutes once the autopsy report came in, and I shared with him some of the report. The surgeon apologized for the fact that my son had died, but he never apologized for the incident itself. Then we never spoke again. He was a sympathetic and gentle man, but over the years I have written to him, I sent him a book that our story was in, and I asked him if he had learned anything, if anything had changed in the way he practiced. That was all I ever wanted to know, and I never heard from him.

I did not want to go the way of litigation, but there was just no other way available to get answers, and I needed to find out if I had done something wrong. At first I could not find a lawyer to take the case because my son was so young, but finally a friend found a lawyer who took the case.

We took sworn depositions from the people involved. I wanted to have it in writing, what had happened to Michael. Ironically, this was a good thing, because one of the emergency room doctors who had recommended the cream for the sores and the swelling said that we were never in the emergency room that day, and there were no records that we had been there. To prove that we were in the emergency room that day I had to go to the pharmacy to show that we had gotten the prescription. Otherwise, there was no proof that this had ever even happened. For this reason alone I was glad that we had gone the route of litigation, so we could have the depositions as evidence. As soon as we finished the depositions I asked the attorney to either settle or drop the case. I did not want to keep going on. So we settled with them.

The Miracles of Medicine

After the lawsuit was finalized I got pregnant again. I had complicated pregnancies with my next two sons, and it became very problematic for me because my past experience with the healthcare system made me distrustful and not the most pleasant patient.

During my last pregnancy, at 20 weeks I started to have a spontaneous miscarriage. Saving the pregnancy meant strict bed rest and stitches to hold the baby in. A wrong move could mean a danger-ously early delivery. At 22 weeks, I felt the unmistakable gush of fluid. My water had broken.

After almost a week in the hospital, a very young doctor came to my room in the hospital. I didn't want him near me because he was too young and too new. But he said to me, "The fluid is gone, the uterus is lying on the baby, and he is probably going to be very deformed. We really have to think about what we are going to do."

We were in a hospital that did not handle high-risk pregnancies, and this doctor asked what we wanted to do and presented us with the risks. It was the first time that anybody had ever made me feel that I was in charge of my care. It was the Thursday evening before Mother's Day weekend. I told him to come back on Monday.

The next morning I went into labor at 23 weeks. The young doctor came back and asked me if I wanted to have the baby there where we knew he would not survive, or if I would like him to try to find a hospital to take me in. I asked to hear a heartbeat. If there was a healthy heartbeat, I wanted him to try. When I heard the heartbeat I told him that I was not going home empty-handed. I learned later that the doctor told the hospital I was 24 weeks pregnant for a better chance that they would take us.

My son was born in the hospital the young doctor sent us to, and I spent almost 5 months in the neonatal intensive care unit with my baby. He had almost every body system fail. He had heart problems, and his lungs weren't developed. He was very sick. The staff encour-aged me to be part of his team and to share my concerns and help care for him. Three times a day and sometimes overnight, I was at his side. Today he is a perfectly healthy teenager in college.

I like to think that I saw the worst in health care and I saw the miracles of medicine. It really started me on the journey of thinking about what people need to know. People should know that they need to be part of the system. In the hospital where my son was in neonatal care, the healthcare professionals, the nurses, and the residents all knew my story. They never shrugged me off or made me feel like a problem. He was actually born in the same hospital where my first son died.

My son came home on oxygen and was on nursing care for 3 years. During this time he needed surgery. The thought of another son having to undergo surgery was traumatic to me, but everyone treated me like an educated parent because this time around I was asking questions. I asked the pediatrician what he would do if it were his child. This wasn't just a surgery; my son had compromised lungs and needed an anesthesiologist who would be comfortable caring for him. I started becoming very assertive, and the communication I had with the staff was good. Because I pursued this in a more educated and assertive manner, I ended up feeling that my son received the best care he could have.

Empowering Patients in New York

During this time I saw on the news that there was legislation pending in New York about getting information on your doctor's background. This struck a chord with me, because while I had been looking for the anesthesiologist and the surgeon for my youngest son's surgery I kept thinking, "Where is the Better Business Bureau for doctors? Where do I search for the background of doctors? Every phone call leads me to another physician-run organization." I did not realize that there was really nothing out there until I saw this news item.

After I saw the report on television, I called the reporter, who gave me the names of the people who were lobbying to get the legislation passed. I began to spend a lot of time in the state capital pushing for the legislation, and I also started going out into communities and doing presentations to help people become more empowered in their care. I would ask the groups where I spoke, "What do you know about your doctor?"

On October 6, 2000, the legislation was signed into law to allow New York patients to get information on their doctors' background. It also gave New York a patient safety center. It was called the New York Patient Health Information and Quality Improvement Act of 2000.

While I was going around speaking in the communities, it seemed that every place I went, everybody had a story. Because of the media attention generated by the legislation, we were able to give out contact information, and people began to call. Within a year I could not handle all the calls, and I went to my congregation in Freeport, Long Island, and asked if we could hold meetings there. We took the name PULSE of NY from the Colorado PULSE group already formed, and we began to have regular monthly support meetings for people who had bad outcomes. Our congregation opened up for the support groups, and they continued for nearly 10 years.

Conclusion

My ultimate goal is that nobody anywhere should ever go to the hospital alone or feel as though they are alone. In the past few years we've taught families in the community to become advocates for each other in a program called Family-Centered Patient Advocacy. We teach family members to be patient safety advocates and to help organize the care of the patient. They learn to understand the complexity of health care, how errors happen, and what needs to be done to avoid medical injury and improve the outcomes. They are not there to replace medical care but to help coordinate it, with a special understanding of safety. All our work is done in collaboration with the people who work in the system.

The other project that we work on is an independent, community-based council called the Patient Safety Advisory Council. The council is made up of different community groups, and I hold focus groups and teach them about patient safety. We have worked with people who are disabled, caregivers for mentally and intellectually challenged children and their families, Hispanic and transgender individuals, pharmacy students, and teenage mothers in shelters. We are always looking for new groups to work with. We use the information these groups give us to create tools to improve their interactions with the healthcare system, with the people who represent these groups empowering them to make change. Together we have developed protocols to help hospitals treat disabled patients safely, we have created a glossary of terms for transgendered patients to share with their physicians, and we have made wallet-sized cards for Spanish-speaking patients with their rights to an interpreter printed on them, to name just a few. There is trust that comes with treating people with dignity. It keeps patients in these groups in the healthcare system by helping them build honest and trusting relationships with their providers.

After my many years of advocacy, the most exciting change I see is that we are finally talking about patient safety. There is so much we can do to help improve involvement and awareness of patient safety for patients, families, and physicians. We want the best. We want patients to excel and do well. There are probably a lot of healthcare providers who wish they knew what some of us know, because this is all we know. There is a whole voice that is missing in patient care and it is definitely the patient.

Case Discussion

Ilene Corina's journey crosses many parts of the healthcare system and illustrates many points, both positive and negative, about medical care in the hospital and the community. Her son Michael died from complications of tonsillectomy and adenoidectomy, an operation whose benefits are not clear in most cases and whose risks are greater than is understood by many members of the public (Mahant et al., 2014). When she was contemplating surgery for Michael, Ilene was not given a balanced assessment of the potential risks and benefits, a process now considered to be required under the principle of shared decision making, in which clinician and patient share information to arrive at a decision based on the best scientific evidence and the patient's own values and preferences (Barry & Edgman-Levitan, 2012). Ilene says she did not know how to choose a doctor and selected her son's surgeon for reasons that had nothing to do with the surgeon's skill or experience. In addition, she says that all discussions of risk with the surgeon were about anesthesia and not about the potential surgical complications that in fact ended up causing her son's death. After Michael's death, the lack of information continued. The surgeon's contact with Ilene was minimal, and she felt forced to turn to litigation for answers.

Ilene visited two emergency rooms and three doctors' offices to seek help for her son as he experienced repeated episodes of bleeding in the week following his surgery. Healthcare professionals in all five locations failed to recognize what in retrospect should have been obvious signs of patient deterioration. Ilene felt that a significant reason for this was failure to listen to her and a desire to downplay her concerns because of their own busy schedules. This lack of regard for the patient's voice was in contrast to Ilene's treatment during the premature birth of her third child, when a young doctor made her aware of her options and went out of his way to help her get the care she had chosen. As a result of her experiences, Ilene worked to help pass medical transparency legislation in New York, and subsequently founded PULSE of NY, an organization whose purpose is to empower patients to work well with their healthcare providers. PULSE of NY now works closely with underserved groups, non-English speakers, and people with special needs.

Questions

1. What do you think are the important criteria for choosing a doctor? What questions should a patient or family member ask? How can the healthcare professional help guide patients through this process?

2. What are the difficulties healthcare professionals may have in presenting a balanced picture of risk and benefit to patients? How might these difficulties be overcome?

3. Many hospitals now have programs that disclose adverse events to families as soon as they happen and provide support for both patients and providers. Research one of these programs and discuss how you think it might have helped in Michael's case.

4. What skills and knowledge does a healthcare professional need to have to provide the sort of compassionate care that Ilene's obstetrician did, even to a patient who might be wary or unreceptive?

5. What do patients need to learn in order to be empowered to get the best care for their family members?

6. Do you think the healthcare system is set up to meet the needs of special needs populations or people who do not speak the national language? What can individual healthcare professionals do to help improve the healthcare interactions of these groups?

7. Which of the core competencies for health professions are most relevant for this case? Why?

References

Barry, M.J., & Edgman-Levitan, S. (2012). Shared decision making—the pinnacle of patient-centered care. *New England Journal of Medicine*, *366*, 780–781.

Mahant, S., Keren, R., Localio, R., Luan, X., Song, L., Shah, S. S., . . . Srivastava, R. (2014). Variation in quality of tonsillectomy perioperative care and revisit rates in children's hospitals. *Pediatrics*, *133*(2), 280–288.

When Healing Harms: Recovering from a Multisystem Traumatic Injury

The Story of Kathy Torpie (New Zealand)

Kathy Torpie

Editors' Note

Kathy Torpie was an active, adventurous, fiercely independent 47-year-old woman in excellent health. In a single unanticipated moment, her life changed forever. One night, on her way home from dinner the headlights of a car driven by a drunk driver traveling at high speed appeared from around the corner in her lane and hit her car, head on.

This is a multifaceted case that spans the continuum of care as a result of a life-threatening traumatic injury. After heroic efforts to save Kathy's life, she underwent dozens of surgeries in the 17 years following the accident, mostly to reconstruct her face and to correct new issues created while trying to correct existing ones. Although there are many stories to tell, Kathy has selected a few vignettes from her journey to highlight how the treatment injuries that she experienced as a patient point to systemic failures that led to unnecessary, often long-term, suffering for her and wasted time and money for the healthcare system.

LEARNING OBJECTIVES

After completing this case study, you will be able to:

1. Discuss essential roles of effective communication.

2. Discuss the importance of developing skills in interprofessional collaboration for health professional training on patient safety in clinical practice.

3. Discuss patient-centered care from the perspectives of patients, families, and health professionals.

4. Describe potential complications and consequences of multitrauma injuries.

The Accident

My accident occurred on a Friday night on a narrow rural road. I was trapped in metal up to my neck while rescuers worked to get me out of the car. I was conscious throughout. I don't recall feeling any pain during this time, but the terror I recall was unspeakable. I was living alone in New Zealand, and my family lived on the other side of the world in the United States. As emergency staff worked frantically to assess my physical injuries, I was terrified and in shock. Once cut from the car, I had to be transferred to a helicopter waiting a few kilometers away in a school parking lot to carry me to the hospital. There I was assessed for my injuries followed by a 12-hour orthopedic surgery undertaken by a senior physician registrar. My left fibula was fractured, and my left tibia and left patella were shattered. My femurs had compound fractures. My left radius and ulna were fractured, several ribs were fractured, both of my lungs were punctured, the hinge of my jaw "snapped like a broken dental plate," and I suffered several bone fractures (La Forte fracture types 1, 2 and 3) in my face. This left me with no bony fragment larger than 1.5 cm intact in my mid face.

The registrar debrided my open wounds, removed my shattered patella, and covered the defect with a muscle flap made from dissecting my left calf muscle. Metal rods were inserted into my left tibia and both femurs, my fractured fibula was aligned, and my left ulna and radius were plated. It was a marathon effort for the registrar and the entire trauma team. He left the final closing up and the surgical notes to another doctor who arrived only shortly before the surgery concluded.

I needed to be transferred within days to a different hospital for plastic surgery to piece together the bony fragments of my facial skeleton with mini plates and screws. The surgical team struggled with the complexity of the damage to my facial structure. It was the second 12-hour surgery in 1 week, and the first of what would amount to numerous other surgical attempts to reconstruct my face over a period of approximately 15 years.

When I woke up in intensive care, I was neither the active nor the independent woman I had been, and I was unlikely to be so again for a very long time, if at all. I was a helpless patient on life support, unable to see, speak, eat, drink, or breathe for myself. I was unable to reach for the call bell. Terrified, confused, and feeling diminished, I found myself trapped in a broken body in an alien environment that spoke in a language I didn't understand. I was totally dependent for even my most basic needs on strangers who knew me only as the "multitrauma" patient.

Vignette 1: Failure to Keep an Open Wound Clean

During the 12-hour plastic surgery to unite the multiple fractures of my facial skeleton, the surgeon was tasked with applying a skin graft to a deep open wound above my left tibia. He discovered that the wound was "quite dirty" and felt that it was unsafe to leave the internal rod in place under the circumstances. He had to call in a more senior orthopedic registrar physician for unscheduled surgery to remove the internal rod and replace it with external metal fixation.

With external fixation now in place instead of the internal metal rod, I would not be able to begin non-weight-bearing rehabilitation in the pool as planned. I was told that I would have to remain in bed for at least a further 6 weeks before any attempt could be made to stand or begin rehabilitation. Making it out of ICU had been a milestone for me. I was excited about beginning rehabilitation and motivated to work hard. The emotional impact of facing a further 6 weeks bedbound, unable to read or watch TV due to double vision, was devastating to me. My time spent in hospital was much longer than it would otherwise have been.

Vignette 2: Postoperative Evaluation Overlooked the Surgical Displacement of a Fractured Fibula

The fractured left fibula, which had been correctly aligned following the original orthopedic surgery, was displaced during the process of removing my internal rod and replacing it. Although I later complained to nurses that my left foot rotated to the outside, no mention of my concern was entered in my chart and no formal functional or orthopedic assessment was made. One nurse responded by propping my rotated foot up with a pillow to hold it in place. When I did finally stand for the first time several weeks later, I had to point my left foot outwards to avoid bearing the weight through the outside of my foot and to keep my hips in alignment. I would eventually require orthotics to walk comfortably. I would never again be able to run, jump, navigate a steep step without assistance, or even walk down a steep incline.

Vignette 3: Attempts to Move a Multitrauma Patient

After successful efforts to save my life, I remained in the ICU on life support for 3 weeks before being transferred to the plastic surgery ward. It was a huge milestone. I could now breathe unassisted, see, speak, and drink fluids. I was a motivated, confident patient. I believed that I was through the worst of it. Shortly after my move to the plastic surgery ward, a nurse came into the room to transfer me from the bed to a chair with the assistance of a tall, male student nurse. She carefully explained the process for the transfer to me and to the student nurse before beginning. I was to move to the edge of the bed. The nurse would support my left leg to keep it from bending. The student would bend to allow me to put my right arm across his right shoulder, and he would grip my right hand while placing his left arm around my waist. At the signal, I was to step onto my right leg while the student lifted me gently by the arm and swung me around to the chair. Then the nurse would place a second chair to hold my left leg safely in place.

Although only the fracture of the left leg was visibly obvious from the external fixation, I did not tell the nurse about my other injuries. I assumed that she had read my chart and knew the full extent of my injuries in planning this maneuver. As I put my weight onto my right (also broken) leg and the student began to stand upright taking my weight through my right side (and recently broken ribs), I collapsed in pain with a surprised scream. The student, in panic, stood abruptly to his full height yanking me up by my right arm. X-rays showed that my ribs had not healed. It was assumed that the pain to my shoulder was a rotator cuff injury and unrelated to my broken ribs. No further investigations were made and I was promptly moved from the plastic surgery ward to the orthopedic ward, where I became the responsibility of an orthopedic team. The plastic surgeon came to examine me only one other time in the months that I remained in hospital.

I continued to have pain and limited movement in my shoulder long after I left the hospital. I required physical therapy, specialist evaluation, and cortisone shots. I was advised by a specialist that I would eventually need to have my shoulder replaced but that I should wait as long as possible given the limited life of replacement joints. By the time I had the operation, my bone had degenerated to the extent that it cracked when the surgeon was preparing it to remove it and he had to replace it with the prosthesis—creating a secondary treatment injury. My shoulder is one of the most enduring of my injuries in terms of pain and disability.

Vignette 4: Reassuring the Patient Without Checking Complaints

As soon as I was able to speak, I told everyone I came in contact with that my wrist hurt. For several weeks I complained about the pain in my wrist but no one seem to listen or take action to address my concerns. The nurses changed all the time. I had no idea who, if anyone, was in charge of my case. I was rounded on weekly by a team of two orthopedic consultants and two orthopedic registrars. Also present were a variety of people I assumed to be medical students and nurses, and occasionally the charge nurse.

It was my naive expectation that when I voiced concerns about my condition that they would be recorded and discussed by the entire team prior to the rounds. I told the nurses, the registrar, the physiotherapist, the charge nurse, even the nurse aide. And I told my friends. "My wrist really hurts!" Everyone reassured me. "But I can't even lift my cup of tea!" I insisted. No one checked. I later discovered that no one recorded my concerns in my chart.

Eventually, I asked if maybe I should do exercises to keep my now stiff wrist mobile. Again, without checking, I was told that might not be a bad idea. No one took me seriously and eventually neither did I. I did what I could to keep my wrist mobile and otherwise used my other hand as I was repeatedly advised to do when I complained of the pain.

As my recovery progressed, the orthopedic consultant announced that they planned to graft bone to my not yet fully united tibial fractures and get me back up on two feet. I asked, "How will I be able to bear weight on crutches if I can't even hold a cup of tea?" That was the first time anyone responded to my concerns by checking my wrist. My wrist was broken. My records showed that a broken scaphoid was among the original injuries, and that following my original 12-hour orthopedic surgery my broken scaphoid bone went undetected.

Given the extent of the injuries I presented with on admission, it is understandable how a fracture in a small bone like the scaphoid was overlooked. It is also understandable that the postop radiology reports of my wrist were overlooked during the handover of my care to a second hospital. But the fact that I had complained of the pain for so long to so many different professionals charged with my care and that not one recorded or checked my concerns for several weeks was not something I could understand. As a patient I was a potential diagnostic resource that could alert my caregivers to problems they may not have been aware of. Instead, a cascade of events ensued that had an impact not only on me, but on staff, on hospital resources, and even on other patients.

I faced unnecessary ongoing pain, and the surgery that would finally get me standing and into rehab had to be postponed. In addition, I had to undergo an additional surgery to repair the scaphoid, which meant prolonged recovery time and the need for additional physical therapy. It would take several additional weeks of home help after I got out of hospital to function with this missed injury. At the system level, the hand surgeon's schedule and that of her patients had to be changed. All of this involved added cost for the hospital in time and resources.

The surgeon who repaired my scaphoid found that the bone had degenerated to the extent that it couldn't hold a screw. She bound it with a wire and cut the end of the wire flush to the bone. When I did finally have the tibial bone graft and began to walk, I had to use a forearm crutch with my left arm in a brace. Consequently, I was unable to use my left hand for months after being discharged from the hospital.

Vignette 5: Communication Problems in the Outpatient Environment

I complained to a physician registrar at a follow-up outpatient clinic that I felt a sharp pain whenever I moved my wrist a certain way, "Like a stab of something sharp. I think there's a wire sticking out." The registrar referred to the surgical notes and explained that according to the surgical notes there was no wire protruding: "The surgeon said she cut the wire flush to the bone." Once again I felt that my concerns were being dismissed, and I felt helpless to do anything about it.

Months passed. I still couldn't use my wrist and still required home help. I insisted on a second medical opinion. I brought my x-rays and medical notes to a hand surgeon and explained the problem. He listened and ordered another set of x-rays. When I next saw him, he said "Of course it hurts! You've got a piece of wire sticking into the joint." The bone had retreated as it healed, leaving a wire edge exposed. The wire was removed in day surgery, and after several more weeks of being in a brace and having physical therapy the pain subsided.

Conclusion

Without the skill and effort of all the healthcare professionals who looked after me, I would not be alive today. I have much to be grateful for. Yet, the care I received also caused unnecessary and preventable harm. I directly experienced the healthcare system, in both public and private settings, at almost every level of care—from being a critical care patient on life support to a long-term inpatient, to a hospital outpatient, to a patient receiving community health services, and an elective surgery patient on multiple occasions. I became aware of the cumulative impact that small oversights and communication failures had on patients, as well as on the caregiving system. I eventually wrote a book about my medical and personal journey of recovery in effort to help others and the system learn from my journey (Torpie, 2005). I deliver keynote presentations to healthcare professionals internationally, offering insights from the patient perspective and solutions based on my expertise as a psychologist together with references to medical literature and organizational theory (Torpie, 2012).

Case Discussion

Trauma accounts for a significant proportion of annual deaths worldwide (Kauvar, Lefering, & Wade, 2006). The World Health Organization (WHO) estimates that in 2000 five million people died of injuries, accounting for 9% of global annual mortality. That same year, 12% of the global burden of disease resulted from injury. Over 90% of the world's trauma mortality occurs in low- and middle-income nations, with those in Eastern Europe having the highest rates. Almost 50% of those who die are between 15 and 44 years of age, with males accounting for twice as many deaths as females. Road traffic accounts for the largest proportion, roughly 1.2 million deaths, per year, or 2.1% of overall mortality. An additional 20–50 million people are injured annually in road traffic incidents. Although most of the world's trauma deaths occurs in developing countries, trauma is a significant cause of injury and death in industrialized nations as well. Road traffic accidents, including those involving motor vehicles, motorcycles, and pedestrians, are the most common causes of trauma requiring admission into intensive care.

Kathy suffered from a multitrauma injury; such injuries may be defined as physical insults or injuries occurring simultaneously in several parts of the body. The multitrauma patient has usually sustained multiple traumatic injuries to the body, affecting different organs and body systems. The multitrauma patient may have a head injury, multiple fractures, and injury to the internal organs of the chest or abdomen. The more body systems involved usually indicates more serious illness.

Trauma is usually categorized as blunt or penetrating. Blunt injuries are a type of physical trauma caused by impact or other force applied by a blunt object. It is more difficult to assess and diagnose blunt injuries, because blunt injuries are not usually internal and may not be obvious. The complications of multitrauma injury include:

- *Hemorrhage.* The loss of large amounts of blood can result in shock and death. Other complications can also arise after massive blood transfusions.
- *Multiorgan failure.* Severe hemorrhage and injury to multiple organs increase the risk of multiorgan failure. The patient with multiorgan failure may require dialysis to support the kidneys, mechanical ventilation to support the lungs, and inotropic drugs to support the heart so that blood may be pumped effectively to all the organs of the body.
- *Infection/sepsis.* The presence of open wounds increases the risk of infection.
- *Pain.* It is common for the multitrauma patient to experience pain. Providing the patient with analgesia (pain medication) is an important aspect of looking after the multitrauma patient.

Preventable medical errors cost hundreds of thousands of lives every year. The associated cost in human and economic terms is unacceptable. Less evident or openly examined is the cost of all the apparently "small" oversights and communication failures that can (and often do) lead to harm that, although not catastrophic or immediately obvious, can cause a ripple effect of subsequent consequences. These small harms—which can lead to greater harms and cost the healthcare system millions of extra dollars—are often not picked up.

Questions

The accepted meaning of terms used in improvement initiatives, such as *patient centered* or *patient experience*, differs based on whose criteria are being applied to the term. The same is true when deciding what is important in communication.

1. What are your criteria for patient-centered care?

2. If the patient were someone you loved very much, would your criteria change? How so?

3. Do you think Kathy Torpie's care was patient centered? Why or why not? What would have made it more patient centered?

4. Is listening, checking, and responding to patient or family member worries and recording the process worth the time and effort it takes? What examples can you think of from Kathy's experience? Are there examples you can share from your own experience?

5. Other than collecting and conveying information, what are other essential roles of effective communication? Why is this important?

6. Knowing that communication failures meant to save time can lead to patient harm and can cost much more time than was initially saved, what forces, beliefs, values, and so on make it possible or even probable that these shortcuts will (and do) continue?

7. How do you rate the importance of interpersonal and communication understandings and skills in health professional training and on patient safety in clinical practice?

8. How do you think patients rate the importance of the way that health professionals relate to and communicate with them and their families in the treatment they receive?

9. What strategies can be implemented to ensure that health professionals learn from errors?

10. Which of the core competencies for health professions are most relevant for this case? Why?

References

Kauvar, D. S., Lefering, R., & Wade, C. E. (2006). Impact of hemorrhage on trauma outcome: An overview of epidemiology, clinical presentations, and therapeutic considerations. *Journal of Trauma*, *60*(6 Suppl), S3–S11.

Torpie, K. (2005). *Losing face: A memoir of lost identity and self-discovery.* New Zealand: HarperCollins New Zealand.

Torpie, K. (2012). Speaking in the patient's voice for a quality healthcare experience. Available at: http://www.kathytorpie.com.

Personal and Professional Development

Healthcare professionals must be able to demonstrate the qualities required to sustain lifelong personal and professional growth. Specific competencies within the Personal and Professional Development domain are to:

- Develop the ability to use self-awareness of knowledge, skills, and emotional limitations to engage in appropriate help-seeking behaviors.
- Demonstrate healthy coping mechanisms to respond to stress.
- Manage conflict between personal and professional responsibilities.
- Practice flexibility and maturity in adjusting to change with the capacity to alter one's behavior.
- Demonstrate trustworthiness that makes colleagues feel secure when one is responsible for the care of patients.
- Provide leadership skills that enhance team functioning, the learning environment, and/or the healthcare delivery system.
- Demonstrate self-confidence that puts patients, families, and members of the healthcare team at ease.

- Recognize that ambiguity is part of clinical health care and respond by utilizing appropriate resources in dealing with uncertainty.

This section of the book is unique in that there are no case studies assigned to illustrate elements of the core competency domain. This book of case studies provides a vehicle for Personal and Professional Development, where health professionals "demonstrate the qualities required to sustain lifelong personal and professional growth." Today's professional health workforce is not consistently prepared to provide high-quality health care and ensure patient dignity and safety. One contributing factor to this problem is the absence of a comprehensive and well-integrated system of continuing education in the health professional journal and formation.

One of the key objectives of this book is to raise awareness and stimulate discussion and action around what your healthcare organization, division, or unit can do to improve patient care by improving the attentiveness to patients and their families.

Dr. Leach provides the afterword for *Case Studies in Patient Safety: Foundations for Core Competencies*. David Leach, MD, was the executive director of the Accreditation Council of Graduate Medical Education (ACGME) for 10 years (1997–2007), and he is perhaps responsible more than anyone for the present national focus on the central role of competencies in redesigning medical education. Dr. Leach has emphasized that a workforce of knowledgeable health professionals is critical to the discovery and application of healthcare practices to prevent disease and promote well-being and is the perfect voice of wisdom to highlight the importance of patient stories in professional formation.

Afterword

Personal and Professional Development

David Leach, MD

"Today's world stands in great need of witnesses, not so much of teachers but rather of witnesses. It's not so much about speaking, but rather speaking with our whole lives."

—*Pope Francis, address from St. Peter's Square, May 18, 2013*

The patients and families in this book are witnesses to how the profession is performing, and in these cases we have failed the test. With the profession come promises, some explicit and some implied, but promises nonetheless, and the promises have been broken. Hannah Arendt argues that humans by their very nature are unreliable and that their actions have uncertain effects. These two factors make for unpredictability. In her view, promises offer a stabilizing influence and create the ground for lasting relationships with others; however, "[t]he moment promises lose their character as isolated islands of certainty in an ocean of uncertainty . . . they lose their binding power and the whole enterprise becomes self-defeating" (Arendt, 1998, p. 244).

In the case of medicine, the promises attempt to acknowledge and to some extent offset our vulnerabilities. We promise to first do no harm, to offer competent care and to comfort when cure is not possible, to put what is good for the patient before what is good for the doctor, to discern and tell the truth about the patient's condition, and to offer a practical wisdom in our clinical judgments, a wisdom that integrates the best generalizable science with the particular context of a given case. These stories expose failed promises.

Hannah Arendt also says that promises come with a companion faculty, forgiveness. Good promises plan for the forgiveness that will be needed when the promise is broken (Batalden, 2013). Forgiveness, like promises, should be taken seriously. It can repair human relationships and can help manage the irreversibility of some human actions. In its absence, promises remain vulnerable ideals. Progress has been made on forgiveness in medicine. Best practices such as transparency, disclosure policies, formal apologies, analysis of error, and redesigning safer systems help make forgiveness possible, and in some systems have achieved the status of promises. However, in the cases reported in this book forgiveness is impaired for a variety of reasons, ranging from a lack of truth-telling; failure to acknowledge a problem; unavailability of key parties, thereby disabling dialogue; and a system of structured conversations dominated by legal rather than human concerns.

It is my belief that these witnesses have exposed a flaw in the personal and professional development of some of the doctors, nurses, and others who are the so-called providers of care in the systems described. It is also my belief that with the exception of a few sociopaths, most healthcare workers do not show up to work wondering how they can hurt their patients; they are, by and large, well-intended, competent, and good people marked by the human vulnerabilities we all share. How did things go so wrong?

To use a horticultural metaphor, I think that much of professional development is focused on the production of good foliage (good grades, publications, grants, new techniques and skills, promotions, titles, etc.) and too little attention is focused on the development of solid roots (values, deeply held truths and beliefs, and a much deeper understanding of what it is to be a professional). There is a failure of the system to acknowledge that the development of professional competence is accompanied by a parallel set of activities that foster or impair character development. The so-called "hidden curriculum" is a very effective way of impairing character development.

I favor the word *formation* over that of *education*. Education implies the transfer of information from one to another, whereas formation implies a shaping process. Learners are shaped by the internal and external contexts in which they learn. If the system in which they are shaped cannot reliably deliver good patient care, if they regularly witness unprofessional behaviors, if they are discouraged from telling the truth as they see it, from acts of genuine altruism and from paying deep attention to the context of the patient in addition to the rules of medicine, they will suffer from a weakened character development. They become cynical, and their native instinct to care for patients becomes attenuated.

The witnesses in this book offer a corrective. The stories they tell are so compelling that only the most cynical can dismiss them. Pope Francis is right, the world needs witnesses more than teachers. Stories can move the human heart. Quantitative data is essential to the progress of science; qualitative data is essential to the progress of medicine, which after all, is not a science, but rather a craft and art that uses science. We have to honor rather than diminish the idealism of students. Armed with their own stories and that of their patients they can help the more senior of us reconnect with our own roots. In the words of Parker Palmer (2004) we can learn how "to live divided no more," to no longer act in a way that is incongruent with our deeply held values and those of the profession.

References

Arendt, H. (1998). *The human condition*, Chicago: University of Chicago Press.

Batalden, P. (2013, May). Personal communication.

Palmer, P. (2004). *A hidden wholeness: Journey toward the undivided life.* San Francisco: Jossey-Bass.

Appendix

Recommended List of Core Competencies for Health Professions

1. Patient Care

Provide patient-centered care that is compassionate, appropriate, and effective for the treatment of health problems and the promotion of health.

1.1. Perform all medical, diagnostic, and surgical procedures considered essential for the area of practice.

1.2. Gather essential and accurate information about patients and their conditions through history-taking, physical examination, and the use of laboratory data, imaging, and other tests.

1.3. Organize and prioritize responsibilities to provide care that is safe, effective, and efficient.

1.4. Interpret laboratory data, imaging studies, and other tests required for the area of practice.

1.5. Make informed decisions about diagnostic and therapeutic interventions based on patient information and preferences, up-to-date scientific evidence, and clinical judgment.

1.6. Develop and carry out patient management plans.

1.7. Counsel and educate patients and their families to empower them to participate in their care and enable shared decision making.

1.8. Provide appropriate referral of patients including ensuring continuity of care throughout transitions between providers or settings, and following up on patient progress and outcomes.

1.9. Provide healthcare services to patients, families, and communities aimed at preventing health problems or maintaining health.

1.10. Provide appropriate role modeling.

1.11. Perform supervisory responsibilities commensurate with one's roles, abilities, and qualifications.

2. Knowledge for Practice

Demonstrate knowledge of established and evolving biomedical, clinical, epidemiological, and social-behavioral sciences, as well as the application of this knowledge to patient care.

2.1. Demonstrate an investigatory and analytic approach to clinical situations.

2.2. Apply established and emerging biophysical scientific principles fundamental to health care for patients and populations.

2.3. Apply established and emerging principles of clinical sciences to diagnostic and therapeutic decision making, clinical problem solving, and other aspects of evidence-based health care.

2.4. Apply principles of epidemiological sciences to the identification of health problems, risk factors, treatment strategies, resources, and disease prevention/health promotion efforts for patients and populations.

2.5. Apply principles of social-behavioral sciences to provision of patient care, including assessment of the impact of psychosocial and cultural influences on health, disease, care seeking, care compliance, and barriers to and attitudes toward care.

2.6. Contribute to the creation, dissemination, application, and translation of new healthcare knowledge and practices.

3. **Practice-Based Learning and Improvement**

Demonstrate the ability to investigate and evaluate one's care of patients, to appraise and assimilate scientific evidence, and to continuously improve patient care based on constant self-evaluation and lifelong learning.

3.1. Identify strengths, deficiencies, and limits in one's knowledge and expertise.

3.2. Set learning and improvement goals.

3.3. Identify and perform learning activities that address one's gaps in knowledge, skills, and/or attitudes.

3.4. Systematically analyze practice using quality improvement methods, and implement changes with the goal of practice improvement.

3.5. Incorporate feedback into daily practice.

3.6. Locate, appraise, and assimilate evidence from scientific studies related to patients' health problems.

3.7. Use information technology to optimize learning.

3.8. Participate in the education of patients, families, students, trainees, peers, and other health professionals.

3.9. Obtain and utilize information about individual patients, populations of patients, or communities from which patients are drawn to improve care.

3.10. Continually identify, and implement new knowledge, guidelines, standards, technologies, products, or services that have been demonstrated to improve outcomes.

4. **Interpersonal and Communication Skills**

Demonstrate interpersonal and communication skills that result in the effective exchange of information and collaboration with patients, their families, and health professionals.

4.1. Communicate effectively with patients, families, and the public, as appropriate, across a broad range of socioeconomic and cultural backgrounds.

4.2. Communicate effectively with colleagues within one's profession or specialty, other health professionals, and health-related agencies (see also 7.3).

4.3. Work effectively with others as a member or leader of a healthcare team or other professional group (see also 7.4).

4.4. Act in a consultative role to other health professionals.

4.5. Maintain comprehensive, timely, and legible medical records.

4.6. Demonstrate sensitivity honesty, and compassion in difficult conversations, including those about death, end of life, adverse events, bad news, disclosure of errors, and other sensitive topics.

4.7. Demonstrate insight and understanding about emotions and human responses to emotions that allow one to develop and manage.

5. Professionalism

Demonstrate a commitment to carrying out professional responsibilities and an adherence to ethical principles.

5.1. Demonstrate compassion, integrity, and respect for others.

5.2. Demonstrate responsiveness to patient needs that supersedes self-interest.

5.3. Demonstrate respect for patient privacy and autonomy.

5.4. Demonstrate accountability to patients, society, and the profession.

5.5. Demonstrate sensitivity and responsiveness to a diverse patient population, including but not limited to diversity in gender, age, culture, race, religion, disabilities, and sexual orientation.

5.6. Demonstrate a commitment to ethical principles pertaining to provision or withholding of care, confidentiality, informed consent, and business practices, including compliance with relevant laws, policies, and regulations.

6. Systems-Based Practice

Demonstrate an awareness of and responsiveness to the larger context and system of health care, as well as the ability to call effectively on other resources in the system to provide optimal health care.

6.1. Work effectively in various healthcare delivery settings and systems relevant to one's clinical specialty.

6.2. Coordinate patient care within the healthcare system relevant to one's clinical specialty.

6.3. Incorporate considerations of cost awareness and risk-benefit analysis in patient- and/or population-based care.

6.4. Advocate for quality patient care and optimal patient care systems.

6.5. Participate in identifying system errors and implementing potential systems solutions.

6.6. Perform administrative and practice management responsibilities commensurate with one's role, abilities, and qualifications.

7. Interprofessional Collaboration

Demonstrate the ability to engage in an interprofessional team in a manner that optimizes safe, effective patient- and population-centered care.

7.1. Work with other health professionals to establish and maintain a climate of mutual respect, dignity, diversity, ethical integrity, and trust.

7.2. Use the knowledge of one's own role and the roles of other health professionals to appropriately assess and address the healthcare needs of the patients and populations served.

7.3. Communicate with other health professionals in a responsive and responsible manner that supports the maintenance of health and the treatment of disease in individual patients and populations.

7.4. Participate in different team roles to establish, develop, and continuously enhance interprofessional teams to provide patient- and population-centered care that is safe, timely, efficient, effective, and equitable.

8. Personal and Professional Development

Demonstrate the qualities required to sustain lifelong personal and professional growth.

8.1. Develop the ability to use self-awareness of knowledge, skills, and emotional limitations to engage in appropriate help-seeking behaviors.

8.2. Demonstrate healthy coping mechanisms to respond to stress.

8.3. Manage conflict between personal and professional responsibilities.

8.4. Practice flexibility and maturity in adjusting to change with the capacity to alter one's behavior.

8.5. Demonstrate trustworthiness that makes colleagues feel secure when one is responsible for the care of patients.

8.6. Provide leadership skills that enhance team functioning, the learning environment, and/or the healthcare delivery system.

8.7. Demonstrate self-confidence that puts patients, families, and members of the healthcare team at ease.

8.8. Recognize that ambiguity is part of clinical health care and respond by utilizing appropriate resources in dealing with uncertainty.

Englander, R., Cameron, T., Ballard, A. J., Dodge, J., Bull, J., & Aschenbrener, C. A. (2013). Toward a common taxonomy of competency domains for the health professions and competencies for physicians. *Academic Medicine, 88*, 1088–1094.

Index

Note: Page numbers followed by *b*, *f*, *n*, and *t* indicate material in boxes, figures, footnotes, and tables respectively.

A

accidental fall in hospital
    case study, 129–137
    fatigue, 134
    hospital environmental and human
      factors, 130–132
    interventions for patients, 137
    patient factors for, 130
    poor vision, 133–134
    prevention risk management strategies,
      132
    risk assessment tool for, 134–135, 136*f*,
      137
    risk factors for, 132
activities of daily living (ADLs), 138
acute hemorrhagic necrotizing enterocolitis,
   283
acute myeloid leukemia, 279
    diagnosis of, 279
acute otitis externa in primary care, 254
adenoidectomy, 298
adrenaline, 251
adverse drug reactions, 255
adverse medical event, patients and staff
    after
    case study, 163–172
    clinicians involved in medical error,
      169
    disclosure, 170, 172
    full-disclosure programs, 172
    harmed patients and their families,
      171
    lack of compassion in health care, 168
    medical harm of healthcare
      institutions, 171

    on patients, families, and health
      professionals, 164–166
allergic reactions, 252
allergy-type treatments, 232
American College of Gastrointestinal
   Endoscopy, 81
amnesia, 89
amniotic fluid, 262
anaphylactic reaction, 252
anaphylaxis, 252
anaphylaxis-related deaths, 252–253
antibiotic allergy, 254
APGAR scores, 48
arachnoiditis, 157
Archives of Internal Medicine, 88
arrhythmias, 88, 90
ASD. *See* autism spectrum disorder
atropine, 251
Australian guidelines, 253
autism spectrum disorder (ASD), 101–115
autoimmune syndrome, 232
autopsy, 196–202
autopsy consent form, 202, 203*f*–205*f*

B

best practice characteristics in ID care, 113,
   113*t*–114*t*
bicarb, 238
bilevel positive airway pressure (BiPAP),
   238
biliary sphincterotomy, 80
BiPAP. *See* bilevel positive airway pressure
blood pressure medications, 179
blunt injuries, 318
bone marrow biopsy, 279

Boothman, Richard, 172
brain death, 252
brain stem, insult to, 51–52
bupivacaine, 165

C

cancer
    case study, 177–189
    diagnosis, 278–279
cardiac catheterization, 85
caregivers
    in acute care settings, 112
    awareness, 113t
    ID, 105
cascade effect, 216, 217
case studies
    accidental fall in hospital, 129–137
    adverse medical event, patients and
        staff after, 163–172
    cancer, 177–189
    complex congenital condition, child
        with, 261–271
    drug allergy, 247–258
    enteral tubing misconnection, 231–244
    equivocal birth, 219–227
    failure to rescue, 277–284
    ID, people care for, 101–115
    intractable pain, patient search for
        answers, 153–160
    maternity care, harm in, 63–71
    multisystem traumatic injury, 309–319
    patient safety advocacy, 297–307
    pediatric heart surgery, 47–59
    permanent disability, 209–217
    postsurgical narcotic overdose in
        hospital, 287–295
    routine appendectomy, 15–26
    Staffordshire General Hospital, 29–45,
        31f
    undiagnosed heart rhythm disturbance,
        83–94
    unexpected postsurgical death, soft
        tissue sarcoma, 117–127
    unexplained hospital death, 191–207
Ceclor, 250
cefaclor, 249, 249n, 253–255

central venous catheter, 233
cephalosporin antibiotics, 252, 255
cephalosporin hypersensitivity, 255
cephalosporins, 253
chemotherapy, 278
    types of, 279
chemotherapy-related leukemia, 279
child with heart defects, description, 48–49
chronic back pain, 159
chronic ear infections, 298
clinic medical records, 255
clinical autopsies, 198, 202
clinical decision support system, 257
    degrees of, 250
    use of, 256
clinical software package, problems with
    decision support in, 256–257
closed tubing system, 242
Clostridium difficile, 20
    infection, soft tissue sarcoma, 119–121
Clostridium perfringens bacteria, 274, 283,
    284
Clostridium septicum, 284
Cochrane Review of falls interventions,
    137
communication
    and care management, 109
    with doctor, 80
    doctor–patient, 217
    with health professionals, 273
    ID, 102
    between parents and health care
        providers, 53–54
    with patients, 90
    problems in outpatient environment,
        316
communication skill, 141–142
community-based services, 103
community health services, 316
community pharmacies, 257–258
community projects, 56
community support, ID, 113t
complex congenital condition, child with
    birth, 262–265
    case study, 261–271
    difficulties of diagnosis, 270
    Pierre Robin sequence, 263, 264, 270

routine training for special
circumstances in neonatal
resuscitation, 270
running a patient and family advisory
council, 269, 269*b*
surgeries, 265–266
treatment, 265
unique challenges, 266, 267*b*
continuity of care, 64
lack of, 70–71
corneal damage, 131
court system in medical injury, role of,
200–201
critical care intensive care unit, 76
Cure the NHS, 41–43

D

death certificate, 199, 224
deBronkart, Dave, 185
decision making
errors in, 11
for operation, 6
decision support rule, configuration of, 257
delirium infection, soft tissue sarcoma, 119
Demerol, 289
Department of Health services, 78
diagnostic error, causes of, 94
diagnostic interventions, informed decisions
about, 1
disability action plan, 113*t*
disability awareness, 113*t*
discharge planning, ID, 113*t*
doctor–patient communication, 217
domain, interprofessional and
communication skills, 141–142
drug allergy
aftermath, 252–254
case studies, 247–258
clinical software package, problems
with decision support in, 256–257
community pharmacies, 257–258
consultation, 249–250
data quality, 255
fatal dose, 251–252
oral antibiotic, treatment of otitis
externa with, 254–255

prescription, writing, 250–251
primary care clinic, 248
use of hybrid and paper medical
records, procedures for, 255–256
drug–allergy software utility, 256
drug–disease interaction, 250
drug–drug interaction, 250
dye, 80
dysfunctional medical system, 11

E

e-health movement, 186
e-Patient Dave, 185
ear pain, 249
echocardiogram, 84–85
ECMO machine. *See* extracorporeal
membrane oxygenation machine
electronic medical records, 250
electronic records system, 255
electrophysiologist, 214
electrophysiology test, 85, 86, 89
emergency department (ED)
ID patients, 104–106
at Mercy Hospital, 108–109
endoscopic retrograde
cholangiopancreatography (ERCP), 62,
73
procedure, 74
endoscopy, without oxygen, 34–37
enteral feeding bag, order for, 241
enteral feeding system, 243–244
enteral solution, bag of, 241
enteral tubing misconnection
case studies, 231–244
error, 240–242
frequency of, 243
higher level of care, 238–240
patient health, 232–233
Entonox, 67
epidemiological sciences, principles of, 61
epidural anesthesia, 154, 157
epinephrine, 238
equivocal birth
case study, 219–227
communication with the parents after
birth, 226

confuse the mother's and baby's
heartbeat on fetal monitor, 220–221
death certificate, 224
faulty equipment, 220–221
insensitive behavior on the part of
clinicians, 227
medical problems, 221–222
staph infection, 223
video camera record during birth, 221
ERCP. *See* endoscopic retrograde
cholangiopancreatography
erythromycin allergy, 255
extensive bruising, 19
extracorporeal membrane oxygenation
(ECMO) machine, 51, 51*n*

F

falls risk assessment tools, 137
family advisory council, 269, 269*b*
Family-Centered Patient advocacy program,
305
family satisfaction, factors of, 26
fat injection, 156
fetal monitor strips, 224
flexible services, ID, 114*t*
forensic autopsy, 198, 201, 202
formal falls risk assessment tools, 135
fractured fibula, surgical displacement of, 312

G

gastronomy tube (G-tube), 265
general practitioner (GP), 248
God's Grace Is Sufficient (Parker), 80
Grief Toolbox, 149

H

haloperidol, 105
HCC. *See* Health Care Commission
Health 2.0, 186, 186*n*
health care
cascade effect in, 216, 217
problem in, 81
Health Care Commission (HCC), 44
health management plan, 114*t*
health professional, training levels of, 195
healthcare plans, co-production of, 110

healthcare professional, 1, 61, 229, 273
patients care evaluation, 97
responsibilities, 175
skill and effort of, 316
healthcare providers, training, 12
healthcare quality, indicators of, 26
healthcare services, 2
healthcare system, 69, 113, 316
unexpected postsurgical death, 125–127
heart arrhythmias, 93
heart catheterization, 89
heart, removal of, 201, 206
heart rhythm disturbance, undiagnosed
case studies, 83–94
health of patient, 84–85
heart rhythm disturbance, 87
medics, 87
potassium level problem, 87, 88
review and causes of death, 87–90
standard of care in Texas, 90–92
heartbeats, irregular, 211
hemoglobin (Hb), 24
hemorrhage, 318
holistic approach, ID, 114*t*
homatropine, 134
HONcode of medical ethics, 158
hospice care, 186–187
hospital, accidental fall in
fatigue, 134
hospital environmental and human
factors, 130–132
interventions for patients, 137
patient factors for, 130
poor vision, 133–134
prevention risk management strategies,
132
risk assessment tool for, 134–135, 136*f*,
137
risk factors for, 132
hospital hierarchy, confusion and poor
communication of teaching, 12
hospital policy, 241
hospitalizations
avoidable, 113*t*
guidelines, 114*t*
of ID patients, 105–110
in Lakeview Hospital, 106, 108–110, 111*f*
in Mercy Hospital, 105–106, 107*f*

hospitals, unexplained death, 191–207
human factors problem, 243
human rights, ID, 114*t*
hybrid medical record system, 254, 255
    procedures for use of, 255–256
hybrid patient health record systems, 255

I

Ibilex, 253
ibuprofen, 289
ICU. *See* intensive care unit
ID. *See* intellectual disability
IgE, 252, 252*n*
Ilosone, 253
Imodium, 21
"in-out" urinary catheterization, 9
infection control doctor, 213
infection/sepsis, 318
informed consent
    for autopsy, 201–202
    for heart cath, 85
INR. *See* International Normalized Ratio
integrated services, ID, 114*t*
intellectual disability (ID)
    best practice characteristics in, 113, 113*t*–114*t*
    care for people with, 101–115
    case study, 101–115
    medications, 103–104
    patient behavior, 103–104
    patients, emergency department, 104–105
    patients hospitalizations, 105–110
intensive care unit (ICU), 251
    ID, 106
intensive eye drop therapy, 134, 137
interagency networks, ID, 114*t*
interchangeable Luer lock, 243
International Normalized Ratio (INR), 210–211
International Standard Organization (ISO) standards, 243
Internet, importance of, 185–186
interpersonal skill, 141–142
interprofessional collaboration, 273–275
intractable pain, patient search for answers

availability of medical information on Internet, 160
case study, 153–160
doctors harmful to patients, 154–156
encouraging patients to be informed consumers, 159–160
Internet forums and websites, 155–156
patient information and symptoms, 154–156
surgical consequences, 156–158
intravenous cannula, 16
intravenous tubing, 244
intravenous vancomycin, 24

J

James's Project, 56
Jerry Carswell Memorial Act, 202
Joint Commission survey, 9

K

ketorolac, 7, 10, 192, 193, 199
kidney stone, cause of death, 192, 199
knee replacement, 288–290
knowledge for practice domain, 61–62

L

Lakeview Hospital
    patients hospitalizations in, 106, 108–110, 111*f*
    profile of, 104*b*
laminectomy, 156
laparoscopic approach, 17
Lewis Blackman Chair of Clinical Effectiveness and Patient Safety, 12
Lewis Blackman Hospital Patient Safety Act, 12, 13
licensed healthcare professional, 242
licensed vocational nurse (LVN), 193, 200
LifeFlight, 239
little Miss A-type personality, 182
local primary care clinic, appointment with, 248
long QT syndrome, 88, 89, 94
Louise H. Batz Patient Safety Foundation, 293
LVN. *See* licensed vocational nurse

M

MACRMI, 172
MAME. *See* Mothers Against Medical
Error
maternity care, harm in
case studies, 63–71
consequences for patient, 68–70
continuity of care, 64
medical condition of patient, 64
mild contractions of patient, 65
medical chart, lack of access, 182–183
medical injuries, role of court system in,
200–201
medical problems, 221–222
medical tubing/catheters, errors with,
242–243
Medically Induced Trauma Support
Services (MITSS), 170
medications, 233, 251, 257
blood pressure, 179
warfarin, 210
MedlinePlus, 249*n*2
Mercy Hospital
patients hospitalizations in, 105–106,
107*f*
profile of, 104*b*
methicillin-resistant *Staphylococcus aureas*
(MRSA), 23, 25
minilaparotomy incision, 17
minimally invasive surgical procedure,
complications of, 11
MITSS. *See* Medically Induced Trauma
Support Services
modern healthcare, delivering, 242
morphine, 192
morphine patient-controlled analgesia
(PCA) pump, 17
mortality rates, pediatric cardiac surgery, 57
Mothers Against Medical Error (MAME),
12
MRI, 89
MRSA. *See* methicillin-resistant
Staphylococcus aureas
multidisciplinary approach, ID, 103
multidisciplinary teams, ID, 114*t*
multiorgan failure, 318
multisystem traumatic injury
accident, 310–311

case studies, 309–319
fractured fibula, surgical displacement
of, 312
multitrauma injury, complications of,
318
multitrauma patient, transferring,
312–314
open wound clean, 311–312
outpatient environment,
communication problems in, 316
patient without checking complaints,
reassuring, 314–316
road traffic accidents, 317
multitrauma patient, 311
transferring, 312–314
myocarditis, 90, 91

N

National Council on Potassium in Clinical
Practice, 88
National Health Service (NHS),
Staffordshire General Hospital, 37–38,
41–43
National Institutes of Health, 81
neonatal intensive care unit (NICU), 49
nerve fiber damage, 155
neutropenic enterocolitis, 283–284
New York Patient Health Information and
Quality Improvement Act of 2000, 305
NHS. *See* National Health Service
NICU. *See* neonatal intensive care unit
non-weight-bearing rehabilitation, 312
noninvasive imaging techniques, 81
nonsteroidal anti-inflammatory drug
(NSAID), 7, 11
nursing error, 243

O

obstructive sleep apnea, 102
Ontario Modified Stratified (Sydney
Scoring) Falls Risk Screening Tool, 136*f*
operation, decision making for, 6
oral antibiotic cefaclor, 249
oral antibiotics, 254
treatment of otitis externa with,
254–255
oral medication, 249

orthopedic surgery, 312, 315
otitis externa, diagnosis of, 249
outpatient environment, communication problems in, 316

P

pacemaker, 211
pain, 318
pain medications, 179
pancreatitis, 80, 81
paper medical records, procedures for use of, 255–256
patient and family advisory council, 269, 269b
patient care, domain, 1–2
patient-centered care, 1
    criteria for, 318–319
    soft tissue sarcoma, 125–126
patient certification, maintenance of, 94
patient-controlled analgesia (PCA) pump, 289, 294
    safety, 292–294
patient experiences
    criteria for, 318–319
    measurement and interpretation of, 26
Patient Safety Advisory Council, 305
patient safety advocacy
    case study, 297–307
    communities to help people, 304
    empowering patients, 304–305
    patient information on a doctor's background, 304–305
    risks and benefits of surgery, 306
    shared decision making in helping patients and families, 306–307
    support for patients and providers, 301
patient satisfaction, 26
patient–doctor relationship, 216
patient's medical record, 255
PCICU. See pediatric cardiac intensive care unit
pectus surgery, 6
pediatric cardiac care, 57–58
pediatric cardiac intensive care unit (PCICU), 50
pediatric heart surgery, case study, 47–59
penicillin, 253
penicillin allergy, 255

penicillin hypersensitivity, 255
perforated giant duodenal ulcer, undiagnosed, 11
peripheral intravenous central catheter (PICC), 234, 241
permanent disability, case study, 209–217
person-centered care, 114t
pethidine injections for pain, 20, 23
physical therapy, 214, 215
PICC. See peripheral intravenous central catheter
Pierre Robin sequence, 230, 261, 263, 264, 270
plastic surgery ward, 312, 313
pneumothorax, 51, 53
poor vision, risk of falls, 133–134
postmortem examination/autopsy consent form, 202, 203f–205f
postoperative constipation, 7
postsurgical narcotic overdose in hospital
    case studies, 287–295
    knee replacement, 288–290
    patient-controlled analgesia, 289, 294
    PCA pumps, 289, 292–294
    risks of narcotic and sedative medications, 293, 294
    trouble breathing, 290–292
practice-based learning and improvement, 97–99
premature ventricular contractions (PVCs), 88
preventable medical errors, 318
primary care clinic, 248
primary care involvement, ID, 114t
process mapping, 7
professionalism, 175–176
PVCs. See premature ventricular contractions

Q

QT interval, 88, 89
quality healthcare, soft tissue sarcoma, 125–127

R

rapid response team, 284
referral of patients, appropriate, 2

registered nurse (RN), 193
renal colic, 17
renal failure, deaths by, 196
retrospective chart review of patients, 11
RN. *See* registered nurse
root cause analysis, unexpected postsurgical
    death, soft tissue sarcoma, 123–125
routine appendectomy, case studies, 15–26
routine endoscopic procedure, 74–75
    awareness, 78–79
    case studies, 73–81
    causes of death, 80
    12 hours after pain medication, 75–76

S

safe forcing function design, 257
scar tissue, 157
Scenic Painting, 178–179
Schwartz diagnostic criteria, 88
Sea of Broken Hearts, A (James), 93
"73 Cents," 188
simulation technology, 12
sleep apnea, 212
social-behavioral sciences, principles of, 61
social media, importance of, 185–186
soft tissue sarcoma, unexpected postsurgical
    death
    analyzing the causes of death, 121–122
    case study, 117–127
    Clostridium difficile infection, 119–121
    delirium infection, 119
    fragmentation of healthcare system
        and minimization, 126–127
    healthcare quality, 125–127
    issues in health care system, 126–127
    patient-centered care, 125–126
    review and root cause analysis,
        123–125
    treatment of patient health and death,
        118–121
    trusts in healthcare relationships,
        126–127
software packages, 250
South Carolina Department of Health and
    Environmental Control, 12, 13
sphincterotomy, 81
*Split the Baby: One Child's Journey Through
    Medicine and Law* (Mannix), 56

Staffordshire General Hospital, 30–33
    case study, 29–45, 31*f*
    communication, lack of with patients,
        37–38
    Cure the NHS, 41–43
    furosemide, 40–41
    heart failure, 38–40
    Ward 11, 33–34
    without oxygen, 34–37
stage 4 kidney cancer, 181
    medical chart, lack of access, 182–183
    medical facts, 184–185
standard of care in Texas, 90–92
staph infection, 223
state health department, complaint against,
    284
sulfa-based drugs, 253
surgery, broken ventilator in, 55–56
systems-based practice, 229–230

T

Tarlov cysts, 155–156
    and arachnoiditis website, 158
TENS pain management machine, 280
Texas Medical Board, 76
therapeutic interventions, informed
    decisions about, 1
therapy-related leukemia, 279
thyroid lymphoma diagnosis, 279
tonsillectomy and adenoidectomy, 298
    evidence-based guidelines, 150
    online resource, 149
    partner with patients and families, 151
    patient health, 144
    surgery and postsurgical events for
        patient, 144, 146–149
Toradol, 7, 192, 193, 199
total parenteral nutrition (TPN), 233
total parenteral solution, 241, 242
trauma, 318
triage process, ID patients, 109
trusts in healthcare relationships, 126–127
tubing connections, redesign of, 243
tumors and growths, 180–181
Tylenol suppositories, 146, 148
type A strains of *Clostridium perfringens*, 283
type C strains of *Clostridium perfringens*,
    283

U

UK's National Health Service (NHS), 3
undiagnosed heart rhythm disturbance
    case studies, 83–94
    health of patient, 84–85
    heart rhythm disturbance, 87
    medics, 87
    potassium level problem, 87, 88
    review and causes of death, 87–90
    standard of care in Texas, 90–92
unexpected postsurgical death, soft tissue
    sarcoma
    analysing the causes of death, 121–122
    case study, 117–127
    Clostridium difficile infection, 119–121
    delirium infection, 119
    fragmentation of healthcare system
      and minimization, 126–127
    healthcare quality, 125–127
    issues in health care system, 126–127
    patient-centered care, 125–126
    review and root cause analysis,
      123–125
    treatment of patient health and death,
      118–121
    trusts in healthcare relationships,
      126–127
unexplained hospital death, case study,
    191–207

V

vaginal birth after cesarean section (VBAC),
    70
Vistaril, 289
vital signs of patients, 6–7, 10

W

Walking Through Grief, 149
warfarin, 210
World Health Organization (WHO), 317
world's trauma mortality, 317